ORTHODONTIC DIAGNOSIS

A DENTAL PRACTITIONER HANDBOOK
SERIES EDITED BY DONALD D. DERRICK, D.D.S., L.D.S., R.C.S.

ORTHODONTIC DIAGNOSIS

W. J. B. HOUSTON

F.D.S. R.C.S. Edin., Ph.D., D.ORTH.

Professor of Orthodontics
Royal Dental Hospital of London
School of Dental Surgery

BRISTOL: JOHN WRIGHT & SONS LTD.
1975

ISBN 0 7236 0380 4

PRINTED IN GREAT BRITAIN BY HENRY LING LTD., A SUBSIDIARY OF JOHN WRIGHT & SONS LTD., AT THE DORSET PRESS, DORCHESTER

PREFACE

I⟶ is ten years since a book of this title first appeared in the Dental Practitioner Handbook series under the authorship of Dr. J. S. Beresford. When I was asked to revise it, I felt that the style was so characteristic of its first author that modification by another would not produce a satisfactory result. An entirely new version was decided upon and the opportunity was taken to update the content and to revise the layout.

However, the objectives of the book remain unchanged: to present to undergraduate students and dental practitioners the basis of modern orthodontic diagnosis.

The publication of a text on orthodontic diagnosis without a corresponding section on treatment methods is unusual but has a number of advantages: orthodontic treatment methods vary but the factors to be taken into account in formulating a treatment plan should be common to all systems; and furthermore, this diagnostic procedure should form the basis of the dental examination of any patient.

The advanced diagnostic aids, such as cephalometric radiographs, of the specialist orthodontist are not dealt with in depth for two reasons: firstly because a thorough exposition of the uses and limitations of these methods would have occupied a disproportionate part of the text; and secondly because these aids are not usually available to the general dental practitioner for whom this text was primarily written.

The examination of a patient's facial morphology and function and of the occlusal pattern need take little extra time once experience has been gained. This is time well spent because it should lead to a more adequate appreciation of the patient's dental problems and it can greatly add to the interest of dental practice.

A number of colleagues have made helpful and constructive comments on this work but I cannot mention them all by name. I would particularly like to thank Mr. K. G. Isaacson for his help. Mr. B. J. Webber prepared the models and Mr. K. F. Taylor was responsible for the photography. Finally, I wish to record my appreciation to Miss A. Taylor for her expert secretarial assistance.

January, 1975   W.J.B.H.

CONTENTS

CHAPTER 1

NORMAL OCCLUSION

A DISCUSSION of normal occlusion is an appropriate starting point for a work on orthodontic diagnosis because 'malocclusions' are judged as departures from the 'normal'; and orthodontic treatment is designed to produce a more 'normal' relationship of the teeth.

It is important to distinguish 'normal occlusion' from 'ideal occlusion'. Ideal occlusion is a theoretical concept based on the morphology of the teeth, but it is almost never found in nature and it is not a realistic treatment goal because few patients will have the full complement of 32 teeth in perfect occlusion at the end of ortho-dontic treatment. The value of ideal occlusion is as a theoretical standard by which other occlusions can be judged. Being a theoret-ical concept based on the anatomy of the unworn teeth, ideal occlusion does not take account of the changes that occur with age. In contrast with ideal occlusion, there can be no precise description of normal occlusion. Normal occlusion allows for minor variations from the ideal which are aesthetically and functionally satisfactory. Thus normal occlusion includes slight irregularities of tooth align-ment and relationship. More severe tooth malpositions and mal-relationships between the arches are described as 'malocclusions'.

This rather vague description of the normal may seem unsatis-factory but it is in conformity with other usages of 'normal': it is not possible to specify the limits of normal height or intelligence any more exactly than it is to demarcate the limits of normal occlusion. Because the boundaries between normal occlusion and malocclusion are unclear, it is possible to find disagreement even between experts on the categorization of borderline cases.

FEATURES OF NORMAL OCCLUSION IN THE DECIDUOUS DENTITION

Arch Form and Alignment (Fig. 1a)

The arches are regular in form and all deciduous teeth must be present, of normal form and in correct alignment. Unlike the per-manent dentition, spacings of two types may be present: (1) Spacings between the incisors. (2) So-called 'primate' spacings mesial to the upper canine and distal to the lower canine.

Arch Relationship (Fig. 1b)

The upper arch is wider and longer than the lower. Thus the buccal cusps of the upper molars should overlap the lower molars and the upper incisors should overlap the lower incisors establishing a normal overjet relationship. The overjet in the ideal deciduous dentition

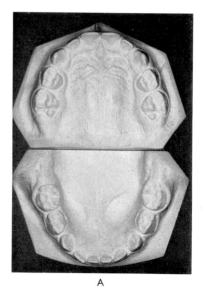

A

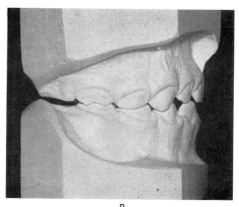

B

Fig. 1.—Normal occlusion in the deciduous dentition.

should be about 2 mm. and the overbite should be about one third of the height of the lower incisor crowns.

Each lower tooth (except for the lower central incisor), should occlude both with the corresponding upper tooth and with the upper tooth in front (*Fig. 1b*). However, because the lower second deciduous molar is longer than the upper the terminal surfaces of the deciduous arches should be flush.

FEATURES OF NORMAL OCCLUSION IN THE PERMANENT DENTITION

Arch Form and Alignment

The arches are regular in form. All teeth must be present, of normal form and in correct alignment. There should be correct approximal contacts between each of the permanent teeth. The permanent incisors, particularly the uppers, are more proclined than the deciduous incisors.

Arch Relationship (Fig. 2)

As in the deciduous dentition, the buccal cusps of the upper cheek teeth should overlap the lowers and the upper incisors should overlap the lower incisors both horizontally (overjet) and vertically (overbite).

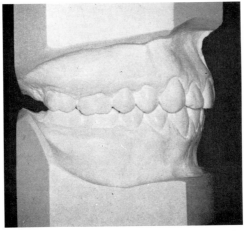

Fig. 2.—Normal occlusion in the permanent dentition.

The lower incisor edges should occlude with the middle part of the palatal surface of the upper incisors. Provided that the angulation between the upper and lower incisors is average, this will ensure a normal overjet and overbite.

Each lower tooth should occlude both with the corresponding upper tooth and, apart from the central incisor, with the upper tooth anterior to it. As in the deciduous dentition, the arches should terminate in the same plane because the lower third molar is longer than the corresponding upper molar.

THE DEVELOPMENT OF NORMAL OCCLUSION

It is important to recognize that there are considerable variations in both the timing and sequence of eruption of the teeth.

The Deciduous Dentition

The upper gum pad is wider than the lower and overlaps it laterally and anteriorly (*Fig. 3*). In the infant the gum pads are rarely brought

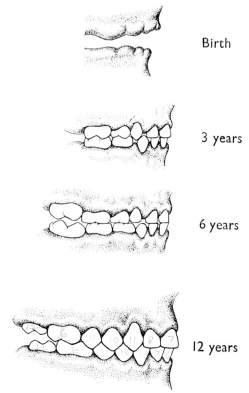

Birth

3 years

6 years

12 years

Fig. 3.—Stages in the development of normal occlusion.

into contact and the tongue lies between them in contact with the lips and cheeks. Deciduous incisors often start to erupt at about 6 months of age and the usual order and times of eruption of the deciduous teeth are indicated in *Table 1*. By the age of 3 years the deciduous dentition should be complete and the features at this stage have already been described.

Changes in the Deciduous Occlusion

Between the ages of 3 and 6 years changes may occur in the deciduous occlusion. These commonly include an increase in intercanine width so that spacing develops or increases between the deciduous incisors and, provided that occlusal wear of the deciduous teeth has flattened

Table 1. TYPICAL AGES OF ERUPTION AND MESIODISTAL WIDTHS OF THE DECIDUOUS TEETH

	Time of eruption in months	Mesiodistal width in mm.
Maxillary Teeth		
Central incisor	8	6·5
Lateral incisor	9	5·0
Canine	18	6·5
First molar	14	7·0
Second molar	24	8·5
Mandibular Teeth		
Central incisor	6	4·0
Lateral incisor	7	4·5
Canine	16	5·5
First molar	12	8·0
Second molar	20	9·5

Note: Eruption times vary considerably—up to 6 months earlier or later than the times given is not unusual. Mesiodistal widths vary by up to 20 per cent on either side of the figures given.

Table 2. TYPICAL AGES OF ERUPTION AND MESIODISTAL WIDTHS OF THE PERMANENT TEETH

	Time of eruption in years	Mesiodistal width in mm.
Maxillary Teeth		
Central incisor	7·5	8·5
Lateral incisor	8·5	6·5
Canine	11·5	8·0
First premolar	10·0	7·0
Second premolar	11·0	6·5
First molar	6·0	10·0
Second molar	12·0	9·5
Mandibular Teeth		
Central incisor	6·5	5·5
Lateral incisor	7·5	6·0
Canine	10·0	7·0
First premolar	10·5	7·0
Second premolar	11·0	7·0
First molar	6·0	11·0
Second molar	12·0	10·5

Note: The figures given both for eruption times and for mesiodistal widths commonly vary by up to 20 per cent on either side of the figures given.

off the cusps and reduced the crown height of the deciduous incisors, the lower arch may move forwards in relation to the upper so that the incisors occlude edge-to-edge (*Fig. 3*). This change in arch relationship reflects a change in dental base relationship due to

5

forwards growth of the mandible in relation to the maxilla. An edge-to-edge incisor relationship is a perfectly normal feature of the late deciduous dentition and should not be mistaken for a mal-occlusion. On the other hand, in some deciduous dentitions there are no occlusal changes during this period.

The Permanent Dentition

The order and timing of eruption of the permanent teeth are indicated in *Table 2*.

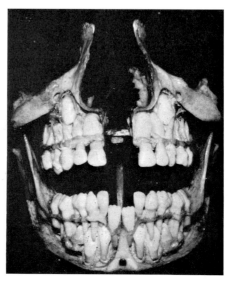

Fig. 4.—Developmental position of the permanent incisors. Note that the permanent incisors develop lingual to the roots of the deciduous incisors and that the permanent upper lateral incisors are overlapped by the central incisors and canines.

THE INCISORS: The permanent incisors are larger than their deciduous predecessors and space is required to accommodate them. This space is obtained by growth in intercanine width and by the fact that the upper permanent incisors, being more proclined, form a larger arc than the deciduous incisors. If there is insufficient space the incisors will erupt crowded. In the upper arch, the lateral incisors may be trapped palatally, reflecting their developmental relationship to the central incisors (*Fig. 4*).

It is common, particularly in the upper arch, for the central incisors to erupt distally inclined so that there is a diastema between them. The lateral incisors also erupt distally inclined (*Fig. 5*). This splayed appearance of the incisors is sometimes called the 'Ugly

6

Duckling stage'. It is important to recognize that this is a normal feature of occlusal development and that the diastema will usually close spontaneously on eruption of the permanent canines.

THE PREMOLARS AND CANINES: Although the permanent canines are wider mesiodistally than their predecessors, the premolars, particularly the second premolars, are narrower than the deciduous molars. The combined width of the permanent canine and premolars is slightly less than that of the deciduous canine and molars. This

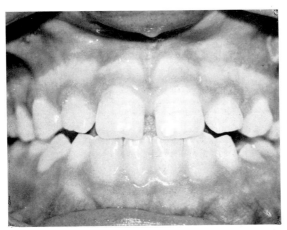

Fig. 5.—The 'Ugly Duckling' stage. The upper incisors are distally inclined and there is a median diastema. This spacing will close naturally on eruption of the permanent canines.

surplus space, which is greater in the lower arch, is known as 'leeway space'. Provided that they are not lost early, the deciduous canines and molars should preserve sufficient space for their successors. However, if deciduous molar teeth, in particular second molars, are lost early or if their contact areas are lost due to caries this space may be reduced by forwards drift of the first permanent molars. This will result in crowding.

THE MOLARS: The first permanent molars should be guided into occlusion by the distal surfaces of the second deciduous molars. If these surfaces are flush (*Fig. 3*) the first molars will erupt cusp-to-cusp. This is a normal relationship in the early mixed dentition. Their correct intercuspation is established on replacement of the deciduous molars by the premolars. The permanent molars drift forwards to take up the leeway space and, as this is greater in the lower arch, the lower molar attains a correct relationship with the upper. The second permanent molars should be guided directly into a correct relationship by the distal surfaces of the first permanent

7

molars. The third molars should follow the same pattern but there is rarely space for them unless other teeth have been extracted.

Changes in the Permanent Occlusion

The most noticeable natural change which occurs in the permanent occlusion between the ages of 15 and 20 years is an increase in lower incisor crowding. The severity of the change varies but it is usually safe to assume that lower incisors which are crowded at 12 or 13 years will be more crowded by 21 years of age. This is largely due to a slight retroclination of the lower incisors which occurs during the later stages of facial maturation. Impaction of lower third molars may contribute by promoting mesial drift of the buccal segments but their influence is usually minor and late crowding occurs even where third molars are absent.

In some cases another change of importance in the permanent occlusion is the forwards movement of the lower arch relative to the upper. This is due to the fact that, on average, the lower jaw grows forwards at a slightly greater rate than the upper face. The occlusal changes are usually small in amount, particularly if there is a good intercuspation of the teeth.

CHAPTER 2
MALOCCLUSION

The boundaries between normal occlusion and malocclusion cannot be drawn precisely. Malocclusion may be defined as those irregularities of the teeth beyond the accepted range of normal. However, the presence of a malocclusion is not in itself justification for treatment. Only if the patient would benefit aesthetically or functionally should treatment be considered. Even then, treatment may not be indicated: the benefits may be trivial; the patient may be unwilling to wear appliances; he may be unsuitable for appliance treatment because of poor oral hygiene and general lack of co-operation. For some malocclusions orthodontic treatment cannot by itself offer a solution and surgery or occlusal rehabilitation may be required as well.

CLASSIFICATION

Malocclusions may involve local irregularities of the teeth or malrelationships of the arches in any of the three planes of space—sagittal, vertical or transverse. For convenience of description it is essential to have a classification. Many classifications of malocclusion have been proposed but only Angle's classification, despite its drawbacks, has withstood the test of time and remains universally recognized.

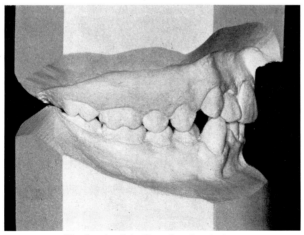

Fig. 6.—Angle's Class I malocclusion.

9

Angle's Classification

Angle's classification is based on arch relationship in the sagittal plane. Angle believed that his classification also provided an index of jaw relationship but it is now recognized that this is not so and the skeletal pattern must be assessed separately (*see* Chapter 4). The key to occlusion in Angle's classification is the relation between the first permanent molars. In normal occlusion (*Fig. 2*) the mesio-buccal cusp of the upper first permanent molar occludes with the anterior buccal groove of the lower first permanent molar.

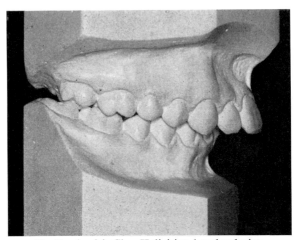

Fig. 7.—Angle's Class II division 1 malocclusion.

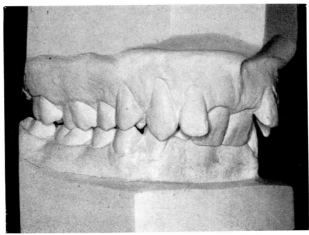

Fig. 8.—Angle's Class II division 2 malocclusion.

Angle's Class I
Malocclusions in which there is a normal anteroposterior arch relationship judged by the first permanent molars (*Fig. 6*).

Angle's Class II
The lower arch is at least one half cusp width distal to the upper, judged by the relationship of the first permanent molars (*Figs. 7* and *8*).

Class II is divided according to the incisor relationship:
DIVISION 1: The upper central incisors are proclined so that there is an increase in overjet (*Fig. 7*).
DIVISION 2: The upper central incisors are retroclined (*Fig. 8*). Characteristically the lateral incisors may be proclined and the overbite is deep. The overjet may be average or increased by only a small amount.

Angle's Class III
The lower arch is at least one half cusp width mesial to the upper, judged by the first molar relationship (*Fig. 9*).

The drawbacks to Angle's classification are evident. The first permanent molars may be missing. They may have drifted following

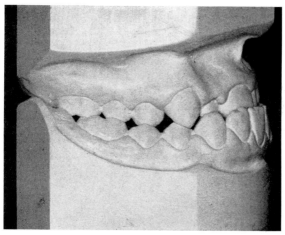

Fig. 9.—Angle's Class III malocclusion.

early loss of deciduous teeth and have to be mentally repositioned before classification—an obvious source of error. The molar relationship may differ between sides. Account is taken only of sagittal arch relationships.

11

Because the molar relationship may be misleading, it is wise to assess the general features of the occlusion and to take into account canine relationships as well when classifying a case. If the canine and molar relationships are not in agreement, the cause for this discrepancy must be sought. Perhaps there has been a drift of a first molar or possibly the canine has been crowded into an incorrect position.

Incisor Classification

Many clinicians find it useful to classify the incisor relationship separately from buccal segment relationship. The incisor relationship may not match the buccal segment relationship and in these cases it is informative to describe both. In addition, a major objective of orthodontic treatment is to establish a normal incisor relationship and it is reasonable that a classification of malocclusion should take this into account. Although Angle's terms are used in classifying incisor relationship, it must be emphasized that this is not Angle's classification.

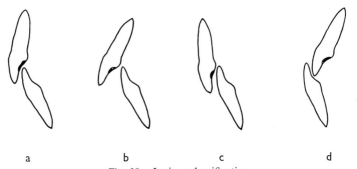

| a | b | c | d |

Fig. 10.—Incisor classification:

   a, Class I.   *b*, Class II division 1.   *c*, Class II division 2.   *d*, Class III.

Class I
The lower incisor edges occlude with the middle part of the palatal surface of the upper incisors (*Fig. 10a*) or lie directly below them if the overbite is incomplete.
Class II
The lower incisor edges lie posterior to the middle part of the palatal surface of the upper incisors.

   Class II incisor relationship is divided into:

> *Division 1:* The upper central incisors
> are proclined (*Fig. 10b*).
> *Division 2:* The upper central incisors
> are retroclined (*Fig. 10c*).

Class III
The lower incisor edges lie anterior to the middle part of the palatal surface of the upper incisors (*Fig. 10d*).

Factors Influencing Incisor Relationship
The overjet is determined partly by the skeletal pattern (p. 31) and partly by the inclination of the incisors (*Fig. 11*). The overbite depends on the incisor classification (*Fig. 10*). If the overjet is normal, the depth of overbite will depend on the angle between upper and lower incisors (*Fig. 12*). The average angle is about 135 degrees. If the inter-incisor angle is much greater than this, the overbite will be deep because the incisors can erupt past one another. When the overjet is increased, the overbite will usually be increased as well unless some other factor, such as a thumb-sucking habit, prevents full eruption of the incisors (*Fig. 12*).

AETIOLOGY OF MALOCCLUSION
The many influences which may prevent the development of a normal occlusion can broadly be divided into 'general factors' and 'local factors'.

General Factors
Include discrepancies between tooth size and arch size, resulting in crowding or spacing, skeletal malrelationships (*see* Chapter 4), and soft tissue factors (*see* Chapter 5).

Local Factors
Result in irregularities of only a few teeth and include:
1. Anomalies in the Number of Teeth
a. EXTRA TEETH: A supernumerary tooth is commonly found close to the midline of the upper arch where it is known as a 'mesiodens' (*Fig. 13*). These teeth are usually peg-shaped or tuberculate and often fail to erupt. They may prevent eruption of, or displace, the permanent central incisors. Where a central incisor fails to erupt or is displaced an intra-oral radiograph should be taken to see if a mesiodens is present. If so it should be removed. Orthodontic treatment may be necessary to align the central incisors.

Extra teeth may be found elsewhere in the mouth. Sometimes, for example in the upper lateral or lower incisor regions, they resemble teeth of the normal series. They will generally cause crowding and have to be extracted.

b. MISSING TEETH: Third molars are commonly missing but this is not a cause of malocclusion. Second premolars or upper lateral incisors (*Fig. 14*) are absent in about 5 per cent of children. Clearly this is of major orthodontic significance and a decision has to be made

13

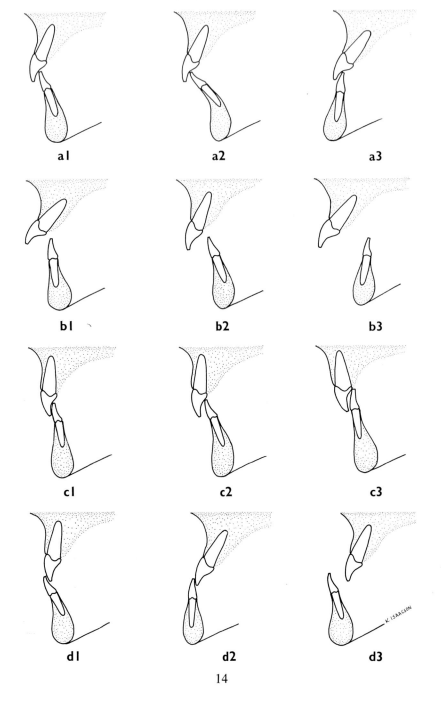

al   a2   a3

b1   b2   b3

c1   c2   c3

dl   d2   d3

whether to close the space or to fit a prosthetic replacement. Because second premolars are so commonly missing (*Fig. 17*, p.21) it is essential to ascertain their presence before extracting other teeth.

c. LOSS OF PERMANENT TEETH: The loss of permanent teeth as a result of trauma, caries or periodontal disease is detrimental to the occlusion. The first molars are the permanent teeth most frequently lost as a result of caries. This can produce a major derangement of the occlusion if the teeth are extracted after the age of 10 years. Space closure, particularly in the lower arch, will be unsatisfactory and the teeth adjacent to the extraction site will tilt. The effects are less unfavourable if the extractions are performed between the ages of 8 and 10 years because in these cases the second molars will erupt further forward and may establish a reasonable approximal contact with the second premolars (*Fig. 15*).

First permanent molars are never the teeth of choice for orthodontic extraction. However, if they are in poor condition before the child is 10 years of age they should be extracted (as soon as possible after 8 years) rather than patched up only to be extracted at a later date with more serious effects on the occlusion. As a general principle, where one first molar has to be extracted before the age of 10 years, the first molar from the opposite side of the same arch should be extracted at the same time. This balancing extraction helps

---

Fig. 11.—Factors determining overjet.

a, A Class I incisor relationship may be produced by:
  1, A Class I skeletal pattern and average incisor inclination.
  2, A Class II skeletal pattern with compensating proclination of the lower incisors.
  3, A Class III skeletal pattern with compensating inclinations of both upper and lower incisors.

b, A Class II division 1 incisor relationship may be produced by:
  1, A Class I skeletal pattern but with proclined upper and/or retroclined lower incisors.
  2, A Class II skeletal pattern with average inclination of upper and lower incisors.
  3, A Class II skeletal pattern with proclination of the upper and retroclination of the lower incisors.

c, A Class II division 2 incisor relationship may be produced by:
  1, A Class I skeletal pattern with retroclined upper and lower incisors.
  2, A Class II skeletal pattern with retroclined upper incisors.
  3, A Class II skeletal pattern with retroclined upper and lower incisors.

d, A Class III incisor relationship may be produced by:
  1, A Class I skeletal pattern with retroclined upper and/or proclined lower incisors.
  2, A Class III skeletal pattern with average inclination of upper incisors and retroclined lower incisors.
  3, A Class III skeletal pattern with average or even proclined lower incisors.

15

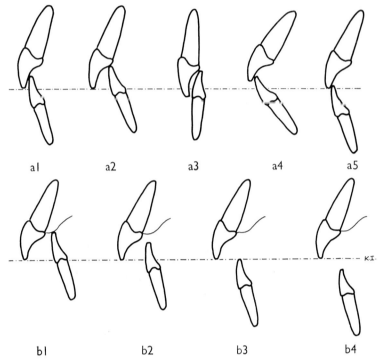

Fig. 12.—Factors determining overbite.

a, Where there is contact between upper and lower incisors the overbite will be:
1, Average if there is a Class I incisor relationship with average inclination of upper and lower incisors.
2, Deep if there is a Class II division 1 incisor relationship.
3, Deep if there is a Class II division 2 incisor relationship.
4, Reduced if there is a Class I incisor relationship with proclined upper and lower incisors.
5, Reduced if there is a Class III incisor relationship.

b, Where there is no contact between upper and lower incisors, and where the overjet is increased the overbite may be:
1, Deep and complete.
2, Deep and only slightly incomplete.
3, Reduced and incomplete.
or 4, There may be no overbite but an anterior open bite.

to preserve the symmetry of the occlusion. It must be emphasized that balancing extraction of first permanent molars should be performed only in the developing dentition where the arch is not spaced and where all other permanent teeth are developing normally.

16

In the lower arch extraction of both first permanent molars between the ages of 8 and 10 years will relieve mild to moderate crowding and will allow a fair approximal contact between the

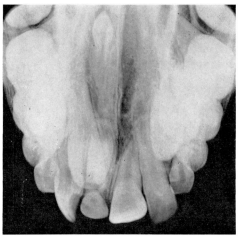

Fig. 13.—One deciduous upper central incisor is retained and a mesiodens is preventing eruption of the permanent upper central incisor. There is another supernumerary tooth in the palate but this has no influence on the incisors.

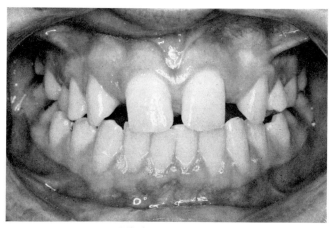

Fig. 14.—Missing upper lateral incisors.

second permanent molar and second premolar. In severely crowded cases the resolution of crowding will not be complete. It is sometimes argued that in these cases the extractions should be postponed until

17

the second permanent molars have erupted so that the appliances can be used to retract the premolars into the extraction spaces. However, this does commit the patient to a considerable period of fixed appliance treatment and is not to be recommended for patients with caries-susceptible mouths.

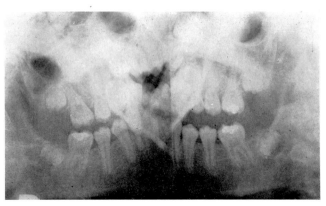

Fig. 15.—All four first permanent molars were extracted at the age of 9 years. At 13 years the second permanent molars have erupted into a reasonable functional position.

In Class I cases with mild crowding, the extraction of the upper first permanent molars at the same time as the lowers will often produce a satisfactory occlusion. However, it is important to recognize that the extraction of lower first permanent molars does not commit one to the extraction of the corresponding upper teeth. If the upper first molars are sound and more space is required in the upper arch, either to relieve crowding or to reduce an overjet, it may be preferable to consider the extraction of first premolars at the appropriate time.

Where the upper first permanent molars have a poor long term prognosis, they can be extracted either early (between 8 and 10 years) or late (after the second permanent molars have erupted). If crowding is mild the teeth should be extracted early. The argument in favour of late removal is that, where more space is required, it is possible to retract the premolars into the extraction space using removable appliances. However, this involves prolonged appliance wear in a patient who is often not ideally suited to orthodontic treatment, and the results are frequently disappointing. There is much to be said, therefore, for extracting upper first permanent molars at an early stage and then treating the case on its merits after the second molars have erupted:

18

   i. Some relief of crowding will have been obtained, and if the patient is not suitable for appliance treatment the occlusion can be accepted.

   ii. If there is mild residual crowding or a slight increase in overjet, extra-oral traction may be used to retract the buccal segments. This is no more time consuming than retraction of premolars and canines following late extraction of first permanent molars, and has the advantage that appliances need only be worn half time.

   iii. If a large amount of space is required it may be necessary to consider the extraction of upper first premolars as well. This may seem radical but it should be remembered that these severe cases could not have been treated satisfactorily by late removal of first permanent molars and extraction of premolars would have been required, whatever the timing of treatment.

d. PREMATURE LOSS OF DECIDUOUS TEETH: This very commonly contributes to the development of a malocclusion but the effects vary greatly and depend in part on—

   i. *The tooth lost:* Early loss of deciduous incisors has little effect on the development of malocclusion. The major effect of early loss of deciduous canines is to improve the alignment of crowded permanent incisors. If the loss is unilateral (sometimes a deciduous canine will be exfoliated due to resorption of its root by a crowded permanent lateral incisor) the midline will shift to the side of loss, producing an asymmetry. For this reason it is wise to balance the loss of one deciduous canine by the extraction of the other deciduous canine in that arch.

      The early loss of first deciduous molars may also temporarily relieve incisor crowding to some extent and, as in the case of the deciduous canine, unilateral loss can produce a shift of centre line. There is also some space loss due to forwards drift of the posterior teeth. Nevertheless, balancing extractions of first deciduous molars should be practised to prevent the development of an asymmetry.

      The major effect of early loss of a second deciduous molar is to allow the first permanent molar to drift forwards (*Fig. 16*), encroaching on space that should have been preserved for the premolars. Because the effects are unpredictable balancing extractions should not be practised.

   ii. *Age of loss:* Clearly, the earlier the deciduous tooth is lost the more pronounced the effects will be.

   iii. *Tooth arch disproportion:* In spaced arches the early loss of deciduous teeth will have little effect. In contrast, where there is crowding or potential crowding, the effect will be more

19

severe. The early loss of deciduous teeth does not create crowding: it merely serves to relocate crowding from the incisor or molar regions to the premolar and canine area. This does not mean that the early loss of deciduous teeth is unimportant because treatment of the crowding may be more difficult following the uncontrolled drift of permanent teeth.

IV. *Intercuspation:* Good intercuspation of the first permanent molars may reduce space loss if there has been early loss of a deciduous tooth in only one arch.

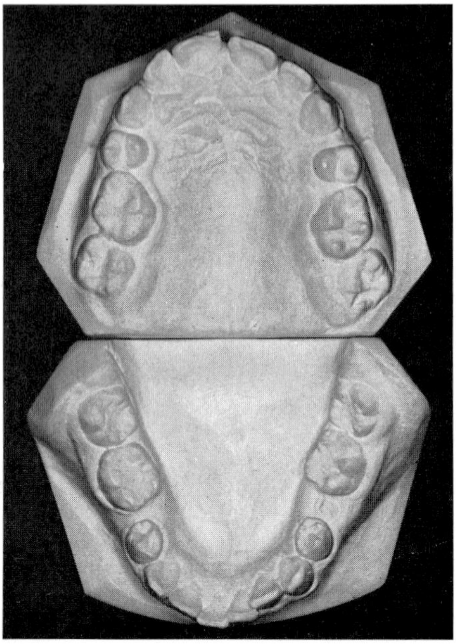

Fig. 16.—Forward drift of first permanent molars following premature extraction of second deciduous molars. The second premolars are crowded as a result.

V. *Space maintainers:* It might be thought that space maintainers should routinely be fitted following the early loss of deciduous teeth. This is not so because—

α. Such mouths are always caries prone and space maintainers are liable to increase food stagnation.

β. Prolonged use of space maintainers may tax the child's good will, so that if orthodontic treatment is necessary at a later stage there may be difficulties with co-operation.

γ. The positive benefits of space maintainers are limited. In crowded mouths orthodontic treatment will be

20

necessary in any case; in spaced mouths, space loss is insignificant.

Only where one or two deciduous molars have been lost from an otherwise good mouth and where it is considered that space preservation will obviate the need for orthodontic treatment should space maintainers be fitted.

e. RETAINED DECIDUOUS TEETH: A deciduous tooth is often retained beyond its normal time of shedding when the permanent successor is absent or misplaced. For example, an upper deciduous canine may be retained when the permanent canine is palatally displaced. However, in some circumstances, retention of the deciduous tooth will in itself prevent eruption of or deflect its successor. For example,

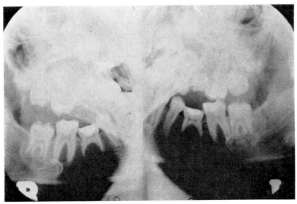

Fig. 17.—Submerging second deciduous molars. Note that the second premolars are absent.

if a deciduous incisor root is not resorbed normally, the permanent incisor will be deflected lingually. Sometimes the roots of a deciduous molar will become ankylosed with the alveolar bone. In the growing child the surrounding teeth and alveolar bone continue to grow in an occlusal direction so that the ankylosed tooth becomes left behind or 'submerged' (*Fig. 17*). A submerging deciduous molar may be associated with the absence of a successor, but if the premolar is present it will be prevented from erupting. Usually the ankylosis is spontaneously resorbed, but if the deciduous molar submerges by more than 2 or 3 mm. it should be extracted with care.

2. *Anomalies in Form and Position of Teeth*

Clearly unusual tooth forms or developmental positions are not compatible with a normal occlusion. Anomalies of form include excessively large teeth, small teeth (e.g. peg-shaped upper lateral incisors) and dilacerated teeth.

Any tooth may develop in an abnormal position although upper permanent canines and third molars are most commonly involved. Other anomalies of position reflecting abnormal developmental positions of the teeth include inversions, transpositions (e.g. the positions of the lower canine and lateral incisor may be reversed) and severe rotations.

3. *Habits*

The habits of orthodontic significance are thumb and finger sucking. The following discussion refers to thumb sucking but the comments apply equally to finger sucking habits.

Thumb sucking does not always have an effect on the occlusion. The magnitude of the effect will depend in part on the frequency of the habit and on the force exerted on the teeth. Thumb sucking is very common in young infants and may at that stage be regarded as normal behaviour. While if the habit persists into the deciduous dentition stage a malocclusion may be produced, this is not usually considered to be of long term orthodontic significance and treatment to stop the habit is not indicated. The effects on the deciduous occlusion may include:

a.   Proclination of the upper and retroclination of the lower incisors

b.   Reduction of the overbite which will be incomplete

c.   Narrowing of the upper arch to match the width of the lower. This necessitates a lateral displacement of the mandible (*see* Chapter 6) to obtain a position of maximum intercuspation. It should be noted that unless there is extensive occlusal wear of the deciduous teeth this displacement will persist into the mixed dentition, so that the crossbite and displacement are perpetuated. Nevertheless, treatment is better left until the child is ready to give up the habit.

The effects of thumb sucking on the relationship of the permanent incisors (*Fig. 18*) are similar to those in the deciduous dentition: namely, an increased overjet and a reduced, incomplete overbite. By the age of 10 years most children are ready to give up the habit. Many do this spontaneously but some require help. If encouragement is not sufficient, a simple removable reminder plate (*Fig. 19*) will often be successful. Following cessation of the habit the incisor relationship may spontaneously improve. If it does not, appliance treatment will be necessary. A unilateral crossbite with lateral displacement of the mandible will not resolve without appliance treatment.

4. *Abnormal Labial Fraenum*

In the infant the upper labial fraenum extends from the inner surface of the lip to the palatine papilla. As the teeth erupt this continuity is lost and the fraenum becomes attached to the labial surface of the

22

alveolar process. Occasionally, the fraenum will persist and this may be associated with a median diastema. In these cases the palatine papilla will blanch if the lip is pulled forwards. In the

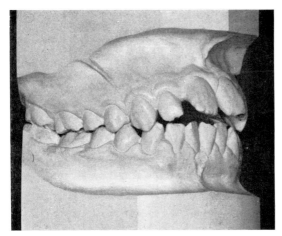

Fig. 18.—A malocclusion associated with thumb sucking.

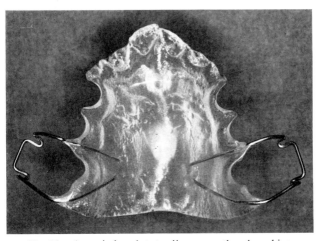

Fig. 19.—A reminder plate to discourage thumb sucking.

majority of cases a median diastema will close spontaneously on eruption of the permanent canines. Rarely, the fraenum is thick and fleshy and is a primary cause of the median diastema. In these unusual cases, a fraenectomy is indicated. Appliance treatment may then be required to close the diastema.

23

CHAPTER 3

ORTHODONTIC RECORDS

THE records required as an aid to diagnosis are study models and radiographs. Clinical photographs both of the face and the dentition are valuable supplementary records.

STUDY MODELS

Models are of importance both as an aid to diagnosis and as a record of an occlusion which may change naturally with age or due to treatment. Orthodontic study models should show the details of all the erupted teeth and as much of the alveolar process as possible (*Fig. 20*). They must be trimmed symmetrically otherwise the eye

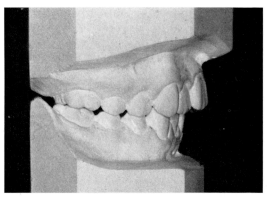

Fig. 20.—Correctly trimmed orthodontic study models. Note that the posterior surfaces are flush so that the models can be correctly articulated by laying them on a flat surface.

will be misled in judging the symmetry of the arch form and they must be occluded correctly and in a reproducible fashion.

Good reference models begin with good impressions. Orthodontic impressions should displace the lips and cheeks so that the full depth of the buccal sulcus is recorded. This 'over-extension' of the impressions is most readily obtained by building up the tray margins with wax or by using special orthodontic trays (*Fig. 21*). The position of maximum occlusion should be recorded by getting the patient to bite through a wafer of softened wax. It is wise to check routinely when the patient attends for diagnosis that models have been correctly articulated.

24

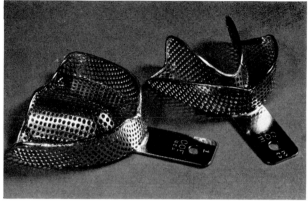

Fig. 21.—Special orthodontic trays. The deep flanges ensure adequate extension of the impressions.

RADIOGRAPHS

Routine Radiographs

Radiographs are required in orthodontic diagnosis to ascertain the presence of unerupted teeth and to monitor the condition of all teeth. Intra-oral films are not satisfactory for this purpose because it can be very difficult to obtain adequate views of unerupted teeth. The most useful films which may be taken with a dental X-ray set are oblique lateral jaw views for all teeth posterior to the canines (*Fig. 22*) and an anterior occlusal view of the upper incisor area (*Fig. 23*). These provide information on all teeth except for the lower incisors. Clinically undetectable anomalies are not common in this area but if there is any doubt, the appropriate intra-oral views should be taken.

Interpretation

Radiographs must be viewed systematically on a properly illuminated screen, otherwise important features can readily be overlooked. It is helpful to have study models available and to identify the teeth on both sets of records.

1. IDENTIFY THE TEETH. Any extra teeth, missing teeth or anomalies of form or position should be noted.
2. EXAMINE THE CROWNS. Although orthodontic views are not well suited to detecting caries, sometimes an approximal cavity which is not visible clinically will be revealed. The crowns of the upper incisors should be examined for deep lingual pits. These will, of course, be visible clinically but they are sometimes much deeper than might at first have been suspected. Lingual pits of this type should be filled prophylactically.

25

Occasionally, a *dens in dente* may be present and the prognosis for the tooth is poor.

The crowns of unerupted teeth should also be examined. Occasionally, the enamel of a second premolar will be hypo-

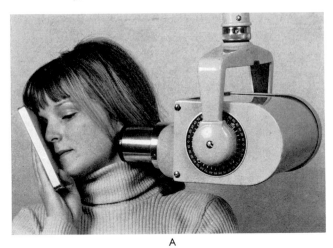

A

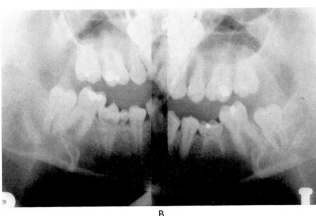

B

Fig. 22.—*a*, Taking an oblique lateral jaw view with a dental X-ray set. The head is rotated towards the side to be radiographed and the tube is directed from just behind the angle of the mandible on the opposite side towards the upper second premolar. The head is rotated to avoid super-imposition of the contralateral side; and tipped back to avoid super-imposition of the cervical vertebrae. The nose should contact the cassette. A fast film with intensifying screens is in the cassette. Special head positioning devices are available.

b, A well taken film shows details of all teeth at least as far forward as the first premolar teeth. It is possible to record both sides on the one film if a lead-rubber flap covering half of the film is attached to the tube side of the cassette. This is moved between exposures.

plastic and this may be detectable on the radiograph (*see Fig. 41*). Clearly if a second premolar is hypoplastic it is not wise to extract another sound tooth as part of orthodontic treatment.

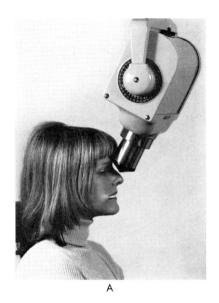

A

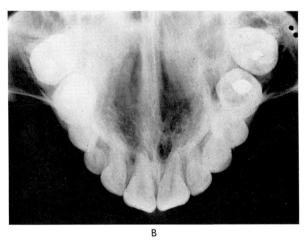

B

Fig. 23.—*a*, Taking an anterior occlusal radiograph.
b, The anterior occlusal radiograph shows the upper incisor teeth, their supporting bone and the anterior part of the palate. It is a good survey view but should not be used for determining the position of erupted teeth. (*See Fig. 25.*)

27

3. EXAMINE THE ROOTS. Any abnormalities of root form should be recorded. Not infrequently idiopathic root resorption affects one or more teeth (*Fig. 24*). If resorption is active it will be accelerated by tooth movement. Furthermore, teeth with short

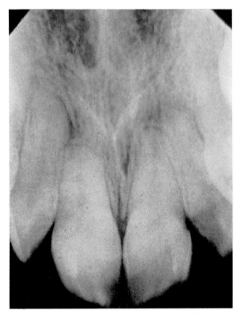

Fig. 24.—Idiopathic root resorption of upper incisors. This patient had not received orthodontic treatment.

roots tip excessively with removable appliances because the fulcrum, which is located close to the middle of the root, is then nearer to the crown of the tooth.

If there is any history of a blow to the upper incisor teeth the roots should be carefully examined for fractures.

4. EXAMINE THE SUPPORTING BONE. A heavily filled tooth may be non-vital and exhibit a periapical radiolucent area. Occasionally areas of sclerosis, cysts or other pathological conditions will be detected.

Supplementary Radiographs

Where the standard views reveal some abnormality it will often be necessary to obtain other views. For example, caries, root resorption or periapical pathology may need to be examined in greater detail on intra-oral films.

28

Parallax Views

Sometimes it is important to ascertain the relationship of an un-erupted tooth, for example a mesiodens or an upper permanent canine which has failed to erupt, to the line of the arch. The anterior

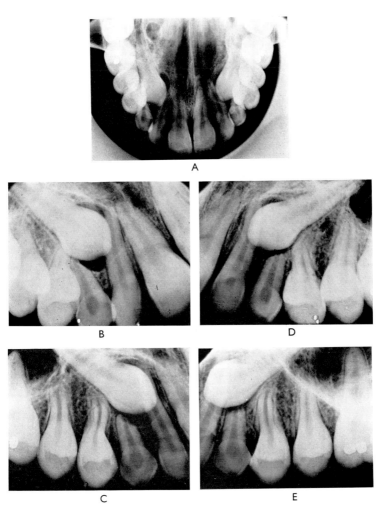

Fig. 25.—Unerupted upper canines often appear to be palatal on an anterior occlusal radiograph. The upper film of each pair (*bc*, *de*) was taken with the tube in a forward position. Note how the root of the lateral incisor appears to move, in relation to the canine crown, in the direction in which the tube was moved. This means that the lateral incisor root is palatal to the canine crown (i.e. the canines are buccal). An anterior occlusal view with one periapical film can be used as a parallax pair.

29

occlusal view gives a distorted picture and most unerupted teeth will appear to be palatal (*Fig. 25*). It is essential in these cases to obtain other films which will permit accurate localization of the unerupted tooth. Parallax views are probably the most convenient to take in the dental surgery. Two periapical films should be taken of the unerupted tooth, the tube being moved about 4 inches between films. Before interpreting parallax films it is important to confirm that they have not been reversed. The tooth which appears to move in the direction in which the tube was moved is palatal (*Fig. 25*).

Where the unerupted tooth is deeply buried, intra-oral films may not give an accurate indication of its height. In general if an unerupted tooth is at or above the height of the apices of the erupted teeth, extra-oral films should be obtained. Lateral skull and posteroanterior skull views are most suitable but cannot be taken with equipment normally available in the dental surgery.

CHAPTER 4

DENTAL BASE RELATIONSHIP

THE dental bases are the bones that support the teeth and alveolar processes, namely the maxilla and mandible. There is no distinct anatomical boundary between the dental base and alveolar process but functionally the alveolar process can be regarded as comprising the bone whose development and presence depends on the presence of the teeth and whose form is influenced by the position of the teeth. When teeth are moved the alveolar process will be remodelled, but the size and position of the dental bases are not affected by the presence of teeth and cannot be altered by normal orthodontic means.

Arch form and size are influenced by dental base form and size, although the orofacial musculature also plays an important part in moulding the form of the arches (*see* Chapter 5). If the dental base is small the teeth will usually be crowded. If the dental base is narrow, the inclination of the teeth may to some extent compensate for this but the arch will still be narrower than average.

Dental base relationships play a fundamental role in determining arch relationships. Three planes of space must be considered: sagittal, vertical and horizontal.

SAGITTAL DENTAL BASE RELATIONSHIPS
(Skeletal Pattern)

The anteroposterior relation of the dental bases is grouped into three classes: Class I where there is a normal relationship of mandible to maxilla, Class II where the mandible is posteriorly placed relative to the maxilla, and Class III where the mandible is prominent relative to the maxilla.

Class I Skeletal Pattern
Ideally the mandible should be slightly less prominent in profile than the maxilla (*Fig. 26*). In this case, provided that the teeth are normally related to the dental bases and the orofacial musculature has produced an average inclination of upper and lower teeth, the upper incisors should overlap the lowers, producing a normal overjet.

A Class I skeletal pattern is frequently associated with a Class I arch relationship. However, it is important to recognize that variations in the position of the teeth on the dental bases or variation in the inclination of the teeth can produce a Class II or a Class III arch or incisor relationship on a Class I skeletal pattern (*see Fig. 11*). Usually these discrepancies in arch relationship are mild and unless

31

other complicating factors are present, the prognosis for orthodontic correction is good.

Class II Skeletal Pattern

Where the mandible is posteriorly placed in relation to the maxilla the skeletal pattern is described as Class II. This will usually be

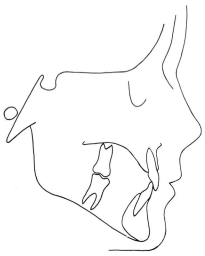

Fig. 26.—A Class I skeletal pattern. The arch relationship is also Class I.

associated with a Class II arch relationship (*Figs. 27* and *28*) although in mild cases the skeletal discrepancy may be compensated for by the inclination of the teeth (*see Fig. 11*). If the skeletal malrelationship is at all severe it will not be possible to obtain a Class I incisor relationship merely by tipping the teeth with simple removable appliances (*see Fig. 45*). The conversion of a Class II division 1 into a Class II division 2 incisor relationship may sometimes produce an aesthetic improvement but it is not likely to benefit the patient from a functional point of view. Fixed appliances are required in these cases in order to obtain a satisfactory result. In the most severe cases it is not possible to obtain a reasonable aesthetic or functional result even with fixed appliance treatment and surgery would be required to treat the skeletal malrelationship.

Class III Skeletal Pattern

Where the mandible is prominent in relation to the maxilla the skeletal pattern is described as Class III (*Fig. 29*). A Class III skeletal pattern is usually associated with a Class III arch relationship. In many Class III cases the inclination of the incisor teeth already compensates to some extent for the skeletal discrepancy, the upper incisors being proclined and the lower incisors retroclined under the influence of the oro-facial musculature. Thus the severity

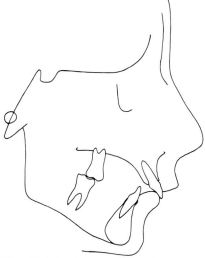

Fig. 27.—A Class II skeletal pattern. There is a Class II divisicn 1 malocclusion.

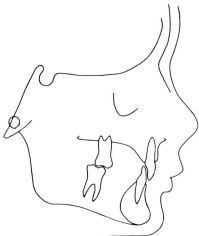

Fig. 28.—A Class II skeletal pattern. There is a Class II division 2 malocclusion.

of the reverse overjet is less than might have been expected from the skeletal pattern. This also means that in many Class III cases the incisor inclination already compensates as much as possible for the skeletal discrepancy and simple orthodontic treatment to correct the incisor relationship is not possible.

Assessment of Skeletal Pattern

The skeletal pattern can be measured on a lateral skull radiograph (*Fig. 30*). Point A is identified on the maxillary profile and the corresponding point (point B) is located on the mandible. The sagittal relationship between these points is measured by the angle ANB (*Fig. 30*). Angles are preferred to linear measurements because in general, angular measurements change little with age. Undue reliance should not be placed on measurements taken from radiographs because, quite apart from the difficulty that sometimes arises in locating point A, the size of angle ANB depends on the position of Nasion as well as on the horizontal relation between points A and B.

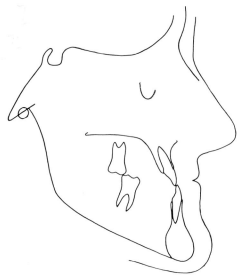

Fig. 29.—A Class III skeletal pattern. There is a Class III malocclusion.

Lateral skull radiographs are rarely available to the dental practitioner. However, it is possible, with experience, to assess the skeletal pattern to quite an acceptable level of accuracy by examining the profile. The patient should sit unsupported with the head in a free postural position so that the Frankfort plane is approximately horizontal, and with the teeth in occlusion. It is important that the correct occlusal position is adopted and that there is no mandibular displacement due to occlusal interference (*see* Chapter 6).

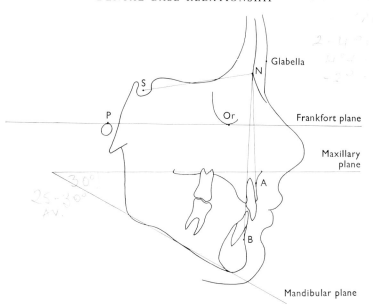

Fig. 30.—Assessment of dental base relationship.

Skeletal Pattern

From this tracing of a lateral skull radiograph, it is apparent that the mandible is slightly posteriorly placed relative to the upper face. The skeletal pattern may be estimated by comparing angles SNA (Sella–Nasion–Point A) and SNB (Sella–Nasion–Point B), which measure the prognathism of maxilla and mandible respectively. The difference between the angles (ANB) gives the skeletal classification:

Angle ANB	Skeletal Classification
between 2 and 4 degrees	I
more than 4 degrees	II
less than 2 degrees	III

In this patient, angle ANB is 5 degrees, indicating a mild Class II skeletal pattern.

Lower Face Height

The heights of mid and lower face should be equal. Mid facial height is measured from glabella (a point between the eyebrows) to the base of the nose; and lower face height from the base of nose to the lower border of chin. In this patient these heights are equal.

Lower face height may also be estimated by the angle between the mandibular plane and either the Frankfort plane or the maxillary plane. The average value for these angles lies between 25 and 30 degrees. If the angle is appreciably greater than this the lower face height is usually large, whereas if the angle is smaller lower face height is reduced.

This patient has a maxillary mandibular planes angle of 28 degrees.

35

There is no difficulty in recognizing severe Class II or Class III skeletal patterns and, with practice, quite accurate assessments can be made. In borderline cases it may be difficult to know whether to classify the profile as Class I or mild Class II, for example, but in such cases the discrepancy is probably so slight as to be of little clinical importance.

It is, of course, the soft tissue profile which is assessed in this way. Although the upper lip is slightly thicker than the lower, the soft tissue profile closely follows the skeletal pattern. If it is considered that lip thickness is misleading the relationship between mandible and maxilla may be examined with the lips retracted, but this will not usually give a more accurate assessment.

It should not be assumed from what has been said above that lateral skull radiographs are unnecessary for the specialist orthodontist. On the contrary, they are an invaluable aid to diagnosis and treatment planning for the patient who requires fixed appliances. However, they are not necessary in general dental practice and considerable skill and experience are required to interpret them reliably.

VERTICAL DENTAL BASE RELATIONSHIPS

The vertical relationship between maxilla and mandible is primarily determined by the shape of the mandible and the resting length of the muscles of mastication. The space between the maxillary and mandibular bases is known as the 'intermaxillary space'. In the child the teeth and alveolar processes develop to establish an occlusion and, as the intermaxillary height increases with growth, vertical growth of the dento-alveolar structures maintains the occlusion.

Where the height of the intermaxillary space is excessive anteriorly, the dento-alveolar structures may reach their full growth potential without achieving an occlusion. In these cases there is a skeletal open bite (*Fig. 31*). It must be emphasized that a skeletal open bite can not be satisfactorily treated by attempting to extrude the anterior teeth which have already grown down as much as possible. Nor should posterior teeth be ground or extracted. This would not affect the resting facial height but would necessitate overclosure to obtain an occlusion. Treatment of this sort will not improve the patient's appearance and the overclosure may result in muscle pain in the long term. Fortunately a skeletal open bite is in itself rarely functionally or aesthetically detrimental. However, a skeletal open bite is frequently present in association with a Class III skeletal pattern. If surgical correction of the skeletal pattern is indicated, the skeletal open bite may be corrected at the same time.

36

Reduction in the height of the intermaxillary space may be associated with a deep overbite but here other factors, such as the occlusion between the incisors, are usually more important.

Assessment of Vertical Dental Base Relationships

The intermaxillary height is often assessed by measuring the angle between the Frankfort and mandibular planes (*Fig. 30*). The average angle is 27 degrees. In general, there is a direct relationship between the anterior height of the intermaxillary space and the Frankfort-mandibular planes angle. However, it is difficult to judge angles by eye with any degree of accuracy. Some form of protractor can be used but errors often creep in.

From a clinical point of view, a simple assessment can be made by comparing the proportions of the lower and middle facial thirds (*Fig. 30*). In the well balanced face these should be equal in height. A relative increase in lower facial height is often associated with a skeletal open bite (*Fig. 31*).

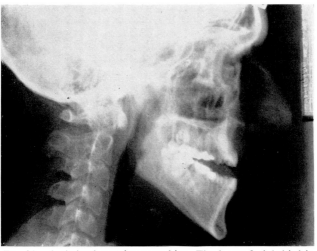

Fig. 31.—A skeletal anterior open bite. The lower facial third is greater in height than the middle facial third. The maxillary mandibular planes angle is also increased.

TRANSVERSE DENTAL BASE RELATIONSHIPS

The width of the dental base has an influence on arch width. In the infant the upper gum pad is wider than the lower and when the deciduous molars erupt the buccal cusps of the upper teeth overlap the buccal cusps of the lower. A similar transverse relationship should be present in the permanent dentition.

Arch width is also influenced by the musculature of the cheeks and tongue. Thus the inclination of the teeth may in some cases compensate for a discrepancy in width between the upper and lower dental bases.

When the upper dental base is narrow in relation to the lower and the inclination of the teeth does not fully compensate for this, the upper and lower arches may be of equal width. In these cases, the mandible will usually be displaced to one side on closure in order to obtain maximum intercuspation (*Fig. 33*, and *see* Chapter 6). This will produce a unilateral crossbite. If there is a still greater discrepancy in dental base width there will be a bilateral crossbite.

Crossbites are particularly common where there is a Class III arch relationship (*Fig. 32*) because a wider part of the mandibular arch opposes a given part of the maxillary arch.

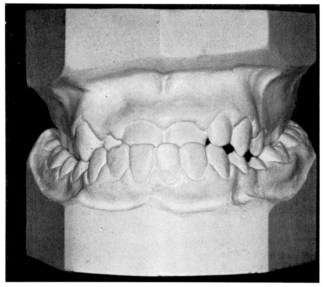

Fig. 32.—A bilateral crossbite.

Occasionally the upper dental base is very much wider than the lower and there may be a lingual crossbite or scissor bite. This is usually unilateral but rarely, in severe cases, it may be bilateral.

Assessment of Transverse Relationships

It is not possible clinically to measure the widths of the dental bases. However, if a crossbite is present it should be remembered that there may be an underlying dental base malrelationship. If the crossbite is unilateral and there is a lateral displacement of the mandible on closure into occlusion, simple expansion will often be successful. A bilateral crossbite reflects a more severe dental base discrepancy and the malocclusion cannot be treated with simple appliances.

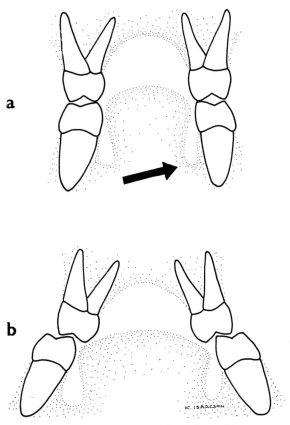

Fig. 33.—Unilateral and bilateral crossbites.

a, In cases with a unilateral crossbite and lateral displacement (indicated by the arrows), the amount of (symmetrical) lateral expansion required in the upper arch is small and the inter-cuspation of the teeth will maintain the correction.

b, In cases of bilateral crossbite there is not a lateral displacement. The amount of simple upper arch expansion required to correct the crossbite would be too great for stability.

CHAPTER 5

SOFT TISSUE MORPHOLOGY AND ACTIVITY

IN orthodontics the soft tissues are the cheeks, the lips and the tongue. Through their form and activity they have an important role in moulding the form of the dental arches. To a large extent the teeth are in a position of balance between the forces of the lips and cheeks and those of the tongue. The forces applied to the teeth by the tongue and circumoral musculature depend in part on the form and position of these tissues and in part on their activity. In most cases, the form and habitual position of the lips and cheeks seem to be more important in determining tooth position than the periodic forces applied by transient muscular activity. Clearly other factors such as the size and relationship of the dental bases influence arch size and form, and occlusal forces play a part in determining individual tooth positions.

It is important to remember that the untreated occlusion is in a state of balance and treatment must be planned to maintain that state or establish another position of balance.

The lower teeth seem to be particularly sensitive to changes in soft tissue balance and it is generally safest to base treatment on preserving lower arch form. Thus it is usually wise to avoid lower arch expansion or a change in the labiolingual position of the lower incisors.

Given normal dental base relationships and soft tissue morphology, if the lower arch is in soft tissue balance and the upper teeth are in correct occlusal relationships with the lower, they too should be in balance. If, however, there is a discrepancy in dental base relationships the position of balance of the upper teeth may be different from that of the lower teeth. For example, if the upper dental base is relatively narrow so that there is a bilateral crossbite (*Fig. 33b*), the upper buccal segments may not be stable if they are expanded to match the lower arch, and they will relapse following appliance treatment. Where the discrepancy is less marked and there is a unilateral crossbite with a lateral displacement of the mandible on closure (*see Fig. 33a*), the amount of expansion required is small and the intercuspation of the teeth may stabilize the result. Similarly, if there is a Class III dental base relationship the upper incisors will be in a position of balance lingual to the lower incisors. Unless there is an overbite so that occlusal forces contribute to their stability

40

(*Fig. 34*), proclination of the upper incisors will be followed by relapse.

Where there is a Class II dental base relationship, the soft tissues may produce a retroclination of the upper incisors to compensate for the dental base discrepancy. This will result in a Class II division 2 incisor relationship (*see Fig. 28*). In other cases, the position of

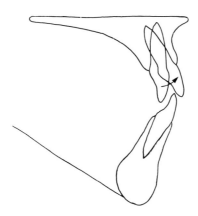

Fig. 34.—Proclination of upper incisors to correct a reverse overjet will be stable only if at the end of treatment there is an overbite. The lower incisors will then hold the upper incisors in the corrected position.

stability of the upper incisors will be further forward so that there is an increase in overjet and a Class II division 1 incisor relationship (*see Fig. 27*). Stability of overjet reduction in these cases depends on finding a new position of soft tissue balance for the upper incisors. This will be obtained if the upper incisors are retracted into a normal relationship with the lower incisors, provided that the patient then maintains a lip seal. It is the relationship of the lower lip to the upper incisors which is the primary factor determining the stability of overjet reduction in Class II division 1 cases (*see Fig. 48*).

LIP FORM

Where the lips are of sufficient length to achieve contact without muscular effort when the mandible is in the rest position they are described as being 'competent' (*Fig. 35a*). If muscular contraction is required to obtain a lip seal the lips are 'incompetent'. Most adults have lips which are either competent or only slightly incompetent but habitually held together with minimal muscular effort. In a small proportion of individuals the height of the lower face exceeds lip length by a considerable amount and so the lips are grossly incompetent (*Fig. 35b*). In these circumstances the lips will be habitually apart. Normally an anterior oral seal is obtained by lip contact, but if there is an increase in overjet or if the lips are grossly incompetent an undue muscular effort would be required to obtain a lip seal and some other mechanism will come into play. Where there is a moderate increase in overjet and if the lips are of adequate length, a forward posture of the mandible will allow a lip seal to be obtained without excessive effort. Should the overjet be large, perhaps associated with a more severe Class II skeletal pattern, an anterior oral seal is more readily obtained by contact between the tongue and lower lip (*Fig. 36*). If the lips are grossly incompetent so that undue muscular effort would be required to obtain a lip seal, then again a tongue-to-lower-lip seal will be produced.

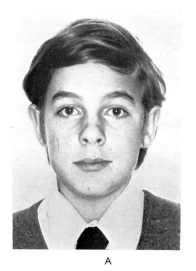 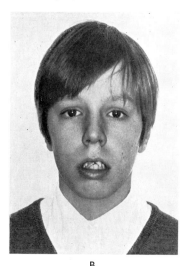

A   B

Fig. 35.—*a*, Competent lips. *b*, Incompetent lips.

These variations in the production of an anterior oral seal are of some clinical importance. The significance of mandibular postures is discussed in Chapter 6. Where a tongue-to-lower-lip seal is adopted, there will usually be a Class II division 1 incisor relationship but the overbite will be incomplete, perhaps by only a very small amount. (The tongue lying over the tips of the lower incisors prevents them from erupting fully.) These patients frequently seek orthodontic treatment for aesthetic reasons. In addition, the gingivae labial to the upper incisors may be hyperplastic as a result of the drying which occurs due to lack of lip cover. This is sometimes incorrectly called a 'mouth breathing gingivitis', but in fact these patients are rarely mouth breathers. There is usually an adaptive anterior oral seal as described above, quite apart from the posterior oral seal formed between the soft palate and the dorsum of the tongue (*Fig. 36*). In planning treatment for this sort of patient it is

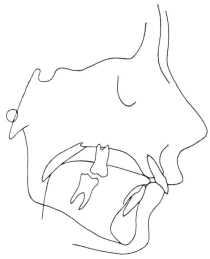

Fig. 36.—An anterior oral seal obtained by contact between tongue and lower lip. There is also a posterior oral seal between the soft palate and dorsum of the tongue.

essential to assess whether or not a lip seal will be readily obtained following retraction of the upper incisors. Most of these patients will quite subconsciously adopt a lip seal on correction of the incisor relationship; the lower lip will be elevated and this will retain the upper incisors in the corrected position. If, however, the lips are grossly incompetent the patient may persist with a tongue-to-lower-lip seal; and the upper incisors, because they are not in muscular balance, will relapse to the original position.

The form of the lips is also important in determining tooth position and it has been suggested by Ballard that the tongue moulds the incisor teeth against the lips. It is certainly true that, given a favour-able dental base relationship, vertically positioned lips are associated with upright incisors (*Fig. 37*) whereas full and everted lips are

43

generally associated with proclination of both upper and lower labial segments (a bimaxillary proclination).

Assessment

Lip form should be examined with the patient sitting in a relaxed position with the mandible at rest and the lips relaxed. Lip activity must be assessed during speech and swallowing. It is often difficult to get the child patient to relax completely. Observations should be made over a period of time, particularly when the patient is not aware that he is being examined—for example as he walks into the surgery or engages in conversation.

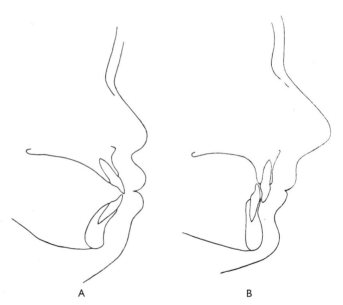

A   B

Fig. 37.—The relationship between lip form and incisor inclination: *a*, full and everted lips associated with a bimaxillary proclination; and *b*, vertical lips associated with a bimaxillary retroclination.

SWALLOWING BEHAVIOUR

Idle swallowing takes place many times in each hour and this repeated activity contributes to the total muscular balance.

The first (oral) phase of normal swallowing is conventionally described as consisting of the following actions: a lip seal is obtained with minimal muscular effort; the tip of the tongue is lightly applied to the palatal mucosa just behind the upper incisor teeth; the teeth are brought lightly into occlusion; the floor of the mouth is elevated by the action of the mylohyoid muscles and the tongue rises to contact the hard palate so that the bolus or liquid is expelled into the pharynx.

That this is too rigid a description is readily ascertained by observing one's own idle swallowing behaviour (although this is difficult to do without modifying the pattern). For example, the teeth may not be brought into occlusion and frequently the dorsum of the tongue is not applied to the hard palate in the manner described. Thus, as might be expected, there is a range of normal variation.

Certain variations of swallowing behaviour do have an orthodontic significance. These may be classified as: (1) adaptive swallowing behaviour; (2) primary atypical swallowing behaviour.

1. *Adaptive Swallowing Behaviour*

Adaptations in swallowing behaviour may occur either because the lips are markedly incompetent or because of anomalies in incisor relationship.

a. Lip Incompetence

As discussed earlier in this Chapter, where the lips are markedly incompetent, an anterior oral seal may be obtained by contact between tongue and lower lip. With the mandible in the rest position, the tongue lies over the tips of the lower incisors. Swallowing may take place with the tongue in this position and with the teeth apart. If the teeth are brought into occlusion during swallowing, the tongue will be contained within the lower arch.

b. Anomalies of Incisor Relationship

i. INCREASE IN OVERJET: Where the overjet is markedly increased, the anterior oral seal will be obtained by tongue-to-lower-lip contact and swallowing will take place as described above. If the overjet is only moderately increased and there is a forward posture of the mandible, idle swallowing will take place with the mandible in this position.

ii. ANTERIOR OPEN BITE OR INCOMPLETE OVERBITE: These may be produced by a number of factors including habits (thumb sucking) and vertical skeletal anomalies (*see* Chapter 4). During swallowing, the tongue will come forwards into the gap. This is a purely adaptive behaviour although it may serve to perpetuate the malocclusion after the primary aetiologic factor has disappeared. For example, the malocclusion caused by thumb sucking does not always spontaneously resolve following cessation of the habit because the adaptive position of the tongue may perpetuate the incisor malrelationship.

45

There is a wide range of adaptations in swallowing, only the most important of which have been mentioned above. Most abnormalities of incisor relationship will necessitate some modification of swallowing behaviour. However, on correction of the malocclusion swallowing anomalies of this type will re-adapt to the new tooth positions. The major diagnostic importance of these variations is that they should be distinguished from the primary atypical pattern of swallowing behaviour which is quite rare but which does have a direct influence on the position of the teeth and which will not adapt to correction of the incisor position.

2. *Primary Atypical Swallowing Behaviour*

Rarely, the tongue is thrust quite forcibly forwards against the palatal surface of the upper incisors during swallowing. This proclines the upper incisors and increases the overjet. The overbite is incomplete. During swallowing there is usually a considerable amount of circumoral contraction.

It is obviously important to recognize a primary atypical swallowing behaviour before beginning orthodontic treatment because the tongue activity will not adapt to a change in position of the upper incisors and relapse will follow.

Assessment

There are no clearcut criteria which enable a confident distinction to be made between a primary atypical swallowing behaviour and an adaptive pattern. Post-treatment relapse is only the proof of a primary tongue thrust.

Certain guide lines can, however, be given:

1. The majority of anomalies in swallowing behaviour are adaptive. In these cases it should be possible to identify the primary factor which necessitates the adaption—for example, grossly incompetent lips, a severe overjet or an incomplete overbite produced by a finger sucking habit.

2. If the overbite is only very slightly incomplete the tongue behaviour is almost certainly adaptive. With a primary tongue thrust, there must be sufficient space for the tongue to protrude over the lower incisors when the posterior teeth are in occlusion. Even in these cases, the underlying factor is probably a habit or an increased lower facial height.

3. With a primary atypical swallowing pattern, the tongue is thrust forwards much more forcibly than with an adaptive behaviour and there is considerable circumoral muscular contraction.

4. Sometimes other features of abnormal tongue control such as lisping are present. However, many children with lisps have perfectly normal swallowing patterns.

46

CHAPTER 6

MANDIBULAR POSITIONS AND PATHS OF CLOSURE

REST POSITION

THE basic position of the mandible in relation to the upper facial skeleton is the rest position. The muscles acting on the mandible are in a relaxed state and the condyles are in retruded unstrained positions in the glenoid fossae. Thus the rest position is essentially determined by the anatomical length of the muscles acting on the mandible. The freeway space is the interocclusal clearance with the mandible in the rest position.

As a working hypothesis it is assumed that the rest position will not change with age or treatment. This assumption is not strictly correct but forms a valid basis for orthodontic treatment. Treatment which is based on the premise that the rest position can be changed, or that it will change with age, will often fail.

Positions of the mandible, such as the rest position, in which the condyles are in a retruded unstrained position are called positions of 'centric relation'. When the teeth occlude in maximum intercuspation the mandible should also be in a position of centric relation.

HABITUAL POSTURES

In the majority of individuals the mandible is in the rest position for most of the time. However, some patients habitually posture the mandible downwards and forwards from the rest position. These postures are usually found in association with certain incisor mal-relationships. Occasionally a patient with a Class II division 1 incisor relationship may posture the mandible deliberately for aesthetic reasons. However, in the majority of cases the posture is subconscious and reflexly maintained. It has been stated by Ballard that these postures are adaptive mechanisms to facilitate a lip seal where there is a moderate increase in overjet. Where a patient can obtain an anterior oral seal by posturing the mandible forwards so that the lips meet more easily this will be done. Such mandibular postures may be associated with three types of incisor relationship: Class II division 1, Class II division 2 and Class III.

In Class II division 1 cases with a moderate increase in overjet, excessive muscular effort could be required to obtain a lip seal with the mandible in the rest position. Provided that lip length is adequate, a forward posture of the mandible allows a lip seal to be obtained

47

with much less total muscular effort. (If the overjet is markedly increased, the anterior oral seal will normally be obtained by contact between tongue and lower lip with the mandible in centric relation, as discussed in Chapter 5.)

In some patients with a Class II division 2 incisor relationship, particularly where the overjet is also increased, a downward and forward posture may also be observed.

In a few patients with a mild Class III incisor relationship, and a normal or increased overbite, the incisors would be in contact, with the mandible in the rest position, and so the mandible is postured slightly forward.

PATHS OF CLOSURE

Ideally the path of closure from the rest position to the position of maximum occlusion should be a simple hinge movement over the two or three millimetres of the freeway space. Two broad groups of exceptions can be distinguished:
1. The path of closure starts from a postured position of the mandible but when the teeth are in maximum occlusion the mandible is in a centric relationship. Here there will be a *deviation* of the mandible during closure.
2. The path of closure starts from the rest position, but due to occlusal disharmonies there is a *displacement* of the mandible.

It is essential to distinguish between deviations and displacements because the treatment will differ. Deviations will not normally be associated with or give rise to pain, faceting of the teeth or periodontal breakdown, whereas displacements may, in the long term, be associated with all three.

Deviations of the Mandible

These are associated with habit postures. Thus with the mandible in the habit position, the inter-occlusal clearance is increased and the condyles are forward in the glenoid fossae. The path of closure is upwards and backwards, but when the teeth are in occlusion the mandible is in a centric relationship (the condyles are in a normal position in the glenoid fossae).

Diagnosis and Treatment

Deviations are most frequently associated with Class II malocclusions where there is an increase in overjet. Habitually the patient will posture the mandible forwards and will maintain a lip seal. When the teeth are brought upwards and backwards into maximum occlusion the mandible will look more retruded and there will be an apparent increase in overjet.

Generally no treatment of the deviation is called for: it will not give rise to muscle or joint pain, nor to periodontal breakdown.

However, if orthodontic treatment is undertaken the patient will lose the habit posture and thus the deviation will disappear at the same time.

Displacements of the Mandible

Premature contacts may necessitate a displacement of the mandible to obtain a position of maximum intercuspation of the teeth. Displacements are frequently long-standing having developed during eruption of the teeth. In some cases the displacement is established in the deciduous dentition, and as the permanent teeth erupt they are guided by occlusal forces into positions that perpetuate the displacement. Displacements can also arise later in life due to uncontrolled drifting of the teeth or loss of posterior support following extractions.

It is important to recognize that when the occlusion has become established considerable adjustment and tooth movement may be required to eliminate the displacement. It is therefore wise to correct occlusal disharmonies at the earliest possible opportunity, preferably during the developing occlusion.

Displacements may either be lateral or sagittal.

LATERAL DISPLACEMENTS are frequently associated with unilateral crossbites. If the maxillary and mandibular arches are of similar widths (*Fig. 38*), a lateral displacement of the mandible is necessary to obtain a position of maximum occlusion and a unilateral crossbite is produced. Lateral displacements are not associated with an increased inter-occlusal clearance nor with overclosure. However, in a proportion of cases muscle pain will develop and will be alleviated only on elimination of the displacement.

The presence of a unilateral crossbite, particularly where the centre lines are not coincident (*Fig. 38*), should arouse suspicions that a lateral displacement may be present. This can be confirmed by carefully observing the patient closing slowly from rest into occlusion. It is helpful to note the relation of the centre lines both with the mandible at rest and in the occlusal position.

Clearly the occlusal interference must be corrected. If there is a unilateral crossbite, symmetrical expansion of the upper arch with an orthodontic appliance is indicated. It should be noted that not all unilateral crossbites are associated with lateral displacements of the mandible: there may be a true asymmetry of the upper or lower arch. If there is no displacement the crossbite will give rise to no functional disability and correction may not be indicated.

SAGITTAL DISPLACEMENTS may arise through premature contacts in the incisor region. In these cases there is sometimes overclosure of the mandible.

49

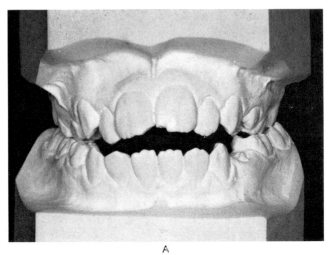

Fig. 38.—Lateral displacement of the mandible associated with a unilateral crossbite. *a*, With the mandible in a position of centric relation, the teeth meet cusp-to-cusp. *b*, In order to obtain a position of maximum occlusion, the mandible is displaced to the left and a unilateral crossbite is produced.

a. Anterior displacements:

i. In the mild Class III case where the incisors meet edge-to-edge, the mandible may be displaced anteriorly to obtain a buccal occlusion (*Fig. 39*). These cases can be diagnosed shortly after the eruption of the upper permanent incisor teeth. It is often suggested that this 'postural Class III' occlusion develops following early loss of deciduous molar teeth, as a result of which the patient overcloses and the lower deciduous canines slide up the cusps of the uppers, enforcing an anterior displacement of the mandible. It should be pointed out that most of these cases have a mild Class III dental base relationship in the first place, although overclosure of the mandible may make this look more severe than it really is (*Fig. 39*). Furthermore, cases of this type can arise where there has been no premature loss of deciduous teeth.

Diagnosis is usually simple. Any patient with a mild reverse overjet and a positive overbite should be examined to determine whether they can with ease bring the incisors into an edge-to-edge relationship. In these circumstances, closure of the mandible to obtain a posterior occlusion is frequently associated with an anterior displacement.

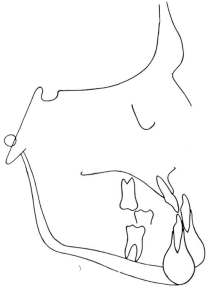

Fig. 39.—With the mandible in centric relation, the incisors meet edge-to-edge but the posterior teeth are out of occlusion. In order to obtain a posterior occlusion the mandible is displaced anteriorly. There is overclosure of the mandible in this case.

An incisor relationship of this type should be corrected ortho-dontically as early as possible. If the malocclusion is left untreated, periodontal damage or muscle pain may develop.

ii. Anterior displacements may also be seen where the upper lateral incisors are instanding and are in lingual occlusion with the lower incisors (*Fig. 40*). The amount of anterior displacement is quite small and these patients do not exhibit overclosure. Unlike the cases described above, the skeletal pattern is Class I or mild Class II. The diagnostic importance is that in the displaced position the

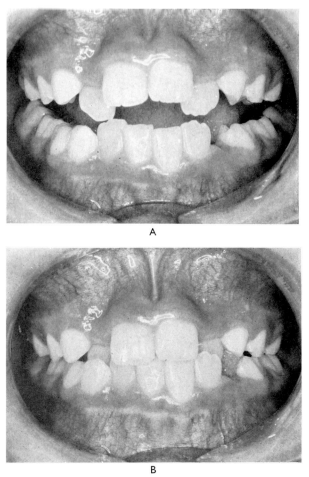

A

B

Fig. 40.—a, With the mandible in centric relation, the lateral incisors meet edge-to-edge with the lower incisors, and the other teeth are out of occlusion.
b, The mandible is displaced anteriorly to obtain maximum occlusion. Notice that this masks the increased overjet on the central incisors.

patient may appear to have a normal overjet on the central incisors. However, on correction of the lateral incisor position an increased overjet will be revealed. In planning orthodontic treatment, sufficient space must be allowed to correct the overjet as well as the lateral incisor position. As with all cases of displacement, the occlusal interference should be corrected early, preferably before the buccal segment occlusion has become established in the displaced position. However, if the upper permanent canine is lying labial to the root of the lateral incisor treatment will have to be delayed until the canine can be retracted.

b. Posterior displacement: It is important to distinguish posterior *deviations* of the mandible, which are quite common in patients with Class II incisor relationships, from posterior *displacements,* which are rare in the intact dentition. Posterior displacements are more often found where there has been loss of posterior support due to extraction of teeth. Such a posterior displacement will often be associated with overclosure and with muscle and joint pain. There may be direct damage to the gingivae palatal to the upper incisors and, in Class II division 2 cases with a deep overbite, labial to the lower incisors. Treatment of these patients involves restoration of posterior support so that both the overclosure and the displacement are corrected.

A small amount of posterior displacement can occasionally be found even when there has been no loss of posterior teeth. This is not usually recognized until symptoms occur in adult life. For these patients careful occlusal analysis followed by occlusal adjustment may be more successful than orthodontic treatment.

CHAPTER 7

INTRA-ORAL EXAMINATION

A CAREFUL intra-oral examination is essential. A hasty, casual or unsystematic inspection is liable to result in oversights and lead to decisions which may have permanent ill effects on the patient's dental health. The clinical examination of the mouth is supplemented by models and radiographs.

1. Teeth Present

Identify the individual teeth, working round each arch. Teeth not present in the mouth should be checked on radiographs. Missing or extra teeth and other abnormalities should be noted. Unless each tooth is positively identified, it is only too easy to overlook things such as an extra lower incisor or a missing second premolar.

2. Condition of Teeth

Teeth with deep carious lesions or extensive restorations should be assessed for long term prognosis. This may influence the choice of teeth for extraction. In children extensive surface decalcification associated with plaque accumulation is not uncommon, particularly on the lingual surface of the lower first permanent molars. The long term prognosis for teeth affected in this way is often poor.

Cingulum pits may be present on the palatal surface of upper incisors. The depth of the pit should be checked on the standard anterior occlusal radiograph (see Chapter 3). As caries leading to pulp exposure can develop rapidly in these pits, they should be filled prophylactically. If an upper incisor is involved with a *dens in dente*, the prognosis may be poor and the tooth may have to be extracted.

Enamel hypoplasia of any teeth should be noted. This may be generalized due to some systemic influence (e.g. long-standing childhood illness) or developmental disorder (e.g. amelogenesis imperfecta). On the other hand, only a single tooth, usually a second premolar, may be hypoplastic (*Fig. 41*). These so-called Turner's teeth are due to interference with formation of the premolar crown, possibly as a result of an acute periapical infection of the deciduous predecessor.

3. Oral Hygiene

The standard of oral hygiene is a good index of the patient's dental awareness and co-operation. Active orthodontic treatment should not be undertaken for the patient with poor oral hygiene, firstly because wearing an appliance when oral hygiene is poor can lead to a rapid deterioration in oral health, and secondly because co-operation will be unsatisfactory.

If oral hygiene is poor instruction should be given and appliance treatment begun only when an acceptable standard is achieved. It is wise to postpone the start of appliance treatment until the patient has maintained good oral hygiene for a reasonable period—say three months.

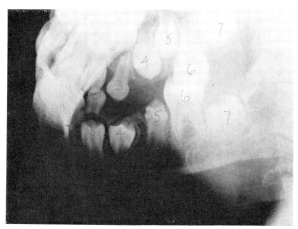

Fig. 41.—A Turner's tooth. When planning extractions, it is important to recognize that the enamel of the unerupted second premolar is hypoplastic.

4. *Periodontal Condition*

In children chronic gingivitis is generally due to poor oral hygiene. Sometimes a hyperplastic gingivitis is present in the upper incisor area. This may be associated with a lack of lip seal and consequent gingival drying. If as a result of orthodontic treatment to reduce an overjet it becomes possible for the child to maintain a lip seal, then the condition will improve. In adults a more detailed periodontal assessment is necessary. The choice of orthodontic extractions may be influenced by the periodontal health. In general, appliance treatment should not be undertaken until the periodontal condition is under control.

5. *Oral Mucosa*

Any dental examination should include an inspection of the cheeks, palate, tongue and floor of the mouth. Lesions of these areas will not usually influence orthodontic treatment unless appliance wear is contra-indicated.

6. Arch Form and Symmetry

Provided that the arch forms are concordant minor variations are not important. Arch asymmetry is of greater significance, particularly if an arch malrelationship results: for example, a buccal crossbite or a discrepancy between centre lines.

7. Crowding and Spacing

A general assessment of the amount of crowding or spacing should be made from study models in order to decide whether extractions will be required. Detailed measurements of space requirements are not very reliable, particularly if some permanent teeth have not yet erupted. If a quantitative estimate of space discrepancy is required it may be obtained as indicated in *Fig. 42*. This measurement does not allow for the space required to correct incisor malrelationships nor to accommodate crowded permanent molars.

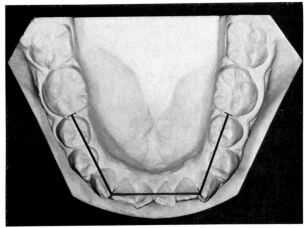

Fig. 42.—Space analysis. The arch perimeter is estimated by taking the linear measurements indicated above. The widths of the erupted teeth are measured directly. The size of unerupted teeth may be estimated from tables of average tooth size or from radiographs.

8. Tooth Positions and Relationships

It is convenient to deal with labial and buccal segments separately. With experience it becomes unnecessary to record in detail the position of every tooth. However, it is important not to overlook any salient feature and some form of systematic examination is essential. Particular attention should be paid to the inclination of the canines and incisors as these are the teeth most frequently involved in orthodontic treatment. If teeth merely need to be tipped into the correct position treatment will be simple and removable appliances may be used, whereas if controlled root movement is required fixed appliances are necessary.

The following details should be recorded:

Labial Segments	Individual tooth malpositions
	Space discrepancy
	Relationships
	Overjet
	Overbite
	Midlines
Buccal Segments	Individual tooth malpositions
	Space discrepancy
	Relationships
	Sagittal
	Vertical
	Transverse

CHAPTER 8

OBJECTIVES OF ORTHODONTIC TREATMENT

THE objective of orthodontic treatment must be to produce an occlusion which is healthy and functionally satisfactory, aesthetically satisfactory and stable.

1. Healthy and functionally satisfactory: There is no evidence that minor irregularities of the teeth or of arch relationship are deleterious to the health of the dentition. However, gross crowding and irregularity probably contribute to and exacerbate peridontal breakdown due to stagnation and abnormal food shedding. Gingival recession may be produced by direct occlusion on the gingivae, or by the traumatic occlusion associated with an instanding incisor (*Fig. 43*). Displacement of the mandible during closure, due to premature contacts can give rise to temporomandibular joint pain.

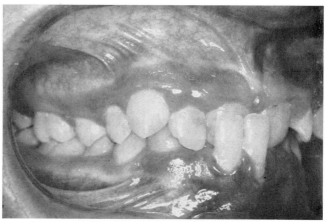

Fig. 43.—Traumatic occlusion. The instanding upper incisors are in a traumatic relationship with the lower central incisors. Such irregularities must be corrected as a matter of urgency.

2. Aesthetically satisfactory: The majority of patients seek orthodontic treatment for aesthetic reasons. A perfect occlusion is generally regarded as aesthetically ideal. However, aesthetic standards cannot be rigidly formulated and not all irregularities of the teeth are aesthetically unsatisfactory. What is acceptable depends on the attitude of the patient himself and on the community in which he lives: for some people a mild element of bimaxillary proclination

is attractive while for others it is unacceptable and is a justification for orthodontic treatment.

3. Stable: The natural occlusion before orthodontic intervention is stable. In planning orthodontic treatment, any change in position of the teeth must be to another position of stability.

These requirements do not imply that the objective in every case must be to produce an ideal occlusion. Indeed, ideal occlusion with 32 teeth in perfect occlusion is a theoretical concept (*see* Chapter 1) which is rarely found in nature and is never produced by orthodontic means. However, many occlusions satisfy the requirements of health, appearance and stability and these may be regarded as 'normal' occlusions.

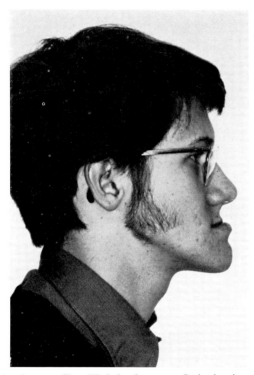

Fig. 44.—A severe Class III skeletal pattern. Orthodontic treatment can by itself do little to improve this patient's facial appearance or occlusal relationship.

While normal occlusion must be the objective of orthodontic treatment, it may not be possible to achieve all the features of normal occlusion in specific individuals. The reasons for this include—

1. Patient unsuitability: the patient may not be willing to wear orthodontic appliances; poor oral hygiene and dental status may preclude appliance treatment; the patient may not be able to attend for regular adjustments.
2. The absence, ectopic position or poor condition of certain teeth may render it impossible to obtain a good result with any sort of appliance.
3. The dental base relationship or soft tissue pattern may be so adverse that it is not possible to produce a satisfactory, stable occlusion by orthodontic means. For example, in cases of gross mandibular protrusion (*Fig. 44*) it is impossible to correct the occlusal relationships by orthodontic means and the poor aesthetic appearance is primarily due to the dental base discrepancy. In some such cases surgery may help to provide a solution, but even with surgery as an adjunct to orthodontic treatment it is not always possible to obtain a normal occlusion.

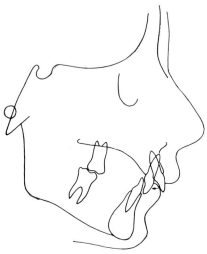

Fig. 45.—Where there is a definite Class II dental base relationship, removable appliance treatment to tip back the upper incisors will merely convert a Class II division 1 malocclusion into a Class II division 2 malocclusion. This will not produce a pleasing aesthetic result and the incisor relationship may become traumatic. In Class II division 1 cases such as this, bodily retraction of the upper incisors using fixed appliances is necessary if a satisfactory result is to be obtained.

4. The skill and experience of the operator is a limiting factor in difficult cases. With some malocclusions a good result can be achieved only by using complex fixed appliances which are

beyond the scope of the dental practitioner and treatment by a specialist is required. However, in many cases such treatment is not available or, even if it is, the patient may not be willing to wear fixed appliances.

In situations where it is not possible to satisfy the requirements of health, appearance and stability by orthodontic means, the decision must be made whether to leave the malocclusion untreated or to accept a compromise result. It must be emphasized that orthodontic treatment should never be undertaken unless it is reasonable to expect that, as a result of treatment, the patient will benefit materially either functionally or aesthetically. The mere conversion of one type of malocclusion into another is no justification for orthodontic treatment. The most difficult decisions have to be made where there is a conflict between the objectives of health, appearance and stability. For example, in certain Class II division 1 malocclusions an improvement in appearance can be achieved only at the expense of health (*Fig. 45*) or stability of the dentition. In some Class II division 2 malocclusions with traumatic overbites it is not possible to produce a stable reduction in overbite without resorting to permanent retention. Where there is a conflict of objectives, preference should be given to health, stability and appearance in that order. However, in some cases the appearance is so unsatisfactory that an aesthetic improvement is of over-riding importance.

CHAPTER 9

TREATMENT PLANNING

MOST active orthodontic treatment is carried out in the late mixed or early permanent dentition. Treatment in the deciduous dentition is not indicated because tooth movement at that stage will have no effect on the occlusion in the permanent dentition. One possible exception is that if cuspal interference leads to a mandibular displacement on closure, treatment to relieve the premature contact may be indicated.

THE EARLY MIXED DENTITION

This stage extends from the eruption of the first permanent molars until eruption of the first premolars. Comprehensive treatment planning cannot be undertaken as an appreciable amount of facial growth still has to take place and the positions and inclinations of many teeth cannot be established. However, certain local malocclusions should be treated at this stage. Perhaps more important, the harmful effects of enforced extraction of carious deciduous and permanent molars can be reduced by balancing extractions. This has been discussed in Chapter 2. In addition, serial extractions may be initiated in the early mixed dentition.

Appliance Treatment

Only minor tooth movements that can be rapidly completed, and which will be stable, should be undertaken in the early mixed dentition. The major problem in carrying out more extensive treatment at this early stage is that frequently it cannot be completed until most of the permanent teeth have erupted. Thus appliance treatment might extend over four or more years. This is not good for the patient's oral health and may unduly tax co-operation.

1. *Instanding Upper Incisors*

Where one or both upper permanent central incisors are in lingual occlusion, and where the overbite will be deep enough to hold them in their corrected positions, treatment should be undertaken early. If the condition is left untreated damage to the periodontal support of the lower incisors, which are sometimes in a traumatic relationship (*see Fig. 43*), may result. If the upper lateral incisors are also in lingual occlusion they may be proclined at the same time, subject to the conditions outlined below.

Upper lateral incisors are often instanding due to crowding (*Fig. 46*). This reflects their developmental position. Providing they are corrected at an early stage and there is a sufficient overbite, they may be stable. However, if the crown of the upper permanent canine is lying over the root of the lateral incisor, treatment should be delayed until the canine has erupted and can be retracted. It should be remembered that crowded lateral incisors are often bodily displaced in a palatal direction and can not be satisfactorily corrected with a removable appliance; and that there may be an anterior displacement of the mandible on closure, masking an increase in overjet on the central incisors (*see Fig. 40*).

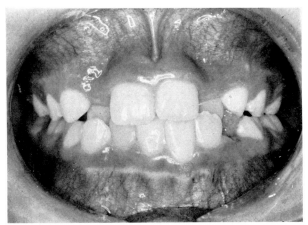

Fig. 46.—Where there is crowding in the upper labial segment the upper lateral incisors may erupt in a palatal position, reflecting their developmental positions.

2. Unilateral Crossbite with a Lateral Displacement of the Mandible

This type of malocclusion should be corrected early by bilateral expansion of the upper arch so that the permanent occlusion does not become established in the displaced position.

Serial Extractions

Serial extraction is a technique where, by the timely removal of certain deciduous and permanent teeth, the attempt is made to relieve crowding and to take advantage of spontaneous tooth movement so that no appliance treatment is required. The full procedure should be limited to Class I malocclusions with crowding and where all teeth are present, sound and in favourable positions.

1. The four deciduous canines are removed as the upper permanent lateral incisors are erupting (at about the age of $8\frac{1}{2}$ years); this should allow the crowded incisors to align spontaneously at the expense of space for the permanent canines.

63

2. About one year later (when the roots of the first premolars have half formed) the first deciduous molars are extracted in order to encourage the eruption of the first premolars in advance of the permanent canines. This is the normal order of eruption in the upper arch, but in the lower arch the canine often erupts first.

3. Finally, when the upper permanent canines are about to erupt, the first premolars are extracted so that the canines, which would be crowded, can erupt into the line of the arch.

If serial extractions are to be performed it must be recognized that a full reassessment should be undertaken at each stage to ensure that this is still the correct plan for the patient. The treatment plan can be altered at any stage if the circumstances change.

The full serial extraction procedure has a number of disadvantages: the child is subjected to extractions on several occasions; the lower permanent canine may erupt in advance of the first premolar so that it becomes impacted between the canine and second deciduous molar, rendering its extraction difficult. Quite frequently the patient requires orthodontic appliance treatment anyway. However, although the classic serial extraction technique is rarely indicated, the principle of timing extractions to take advantage of natural tooth movement is still valid. For example, in carefully selected cases the removal of deciduous canines to allow early spontaneous alignment of crowded incisors may reduce the complexity of later appliance treatment; and the removal of a first premolar before a crowded, mesially inclined canine has fully erupted allows it to drift directly into the extraction space without appliance treatment.

THE LATE MIXED AND PERMANENT DENTITION

Orthodontic treatment is usually undertaken in the late mixed or early permanent dentition because—

1. Most of the permanent teeth have erupted and the amount of crowding and the positions of the teeth can be reliably assessed.

2. Treatment can be completed in an acceptable period of time.

3. Children in this age group are more willing to wear appliances than are older or younger patients.

The principles of treatment planning for adult patients are similar to those described below for the late mixed and early permanent dentition. However, because adults are not willing to wear orthodontic appliances over extended periods of time, treatment should be kept as simple as possible and treatment objectives may have to be limited.

In planning treatment for the patient in the late mixed or early permanent dentition, it must be remembered that the facial skeleton

64

is still growing and that the dental base relationship may change. There is at the present time no method by which the pattern of facial growth for the individual can be reliably predicted and the assumption has to be made that an average growth pattern will be followed: that is that the mandible will grow downwards and forwards slightly faster than the maxilla.

This assumption provides a satisfactory basis for treatment planning in the majority of cases, as changes in the untreated occlusion are usually confined to a slight increase in lower incisor crowding. An unfavourable growth pattern may adversely affect treatment in a few individuals. For example, in some Class III malocclusions more marked forward growth of the mandible may result in failure or relapse of orthodontic treatment. Only broad guidelines to treatment planning can be given here. These principles must be adapted for the individual case in order to cope with local variations in tooth position. It should always be remembered that if removable appliances are used the teeth will be tipped about a point close to the middle of the root. If controlled root movement is required fixed appliances must be used. It is useful to plan treatment first of the lower arch and then of the upper arch so that it conforms to the lower, taking into account limitations which the dental base relationship and soft tissue pattern may impose.

The Lower Arch

It has already been emphasized that lower arch width must be accepted and that the lower incisor position cannot be reliably altered. Treatment planning should therefore be based on the existing form of the lower arch and directed to relief of crowding and correction of individual irregularities.

Clearly, no treatment is indicated for the well aligned lower arch. If, however, there is crowding of a severity sufficient to warrant treatment extractions will have to be considered. Provided that all teeth are present, sound and in favourable positions, the choice of extraction will depend on the site and severity of crowding.

Crowding of the lower incisors or canines is most successfully treated by extraction of first premolars, given canines that are mesially inclined. In the late mixed or early permanent dentition, considerable spontaneous improvement in alignment is to be expected following these extractions, and closure of any residual extraction space will usually occur through forward drift of the buccal segments. Provided that the canines were originally mesially inclined, the approximal contact between the canine and second premolar is usually acceptable. If the lower canines are not mesially inclined a fixed appliance will be necessary to obtain satisfactory alignment.

65

Although it often seems to offer a simple solution to lower arch crowding, the extraction of a lower incisor is to be avoided whenever possible because crowding of the three remaining incisors frequently develops. Furthermore, it can be difficult to obtain a satisfactory arrangement of four upper incisors around three lower.

Crowding in the premolar region, which usually involves the second premolar as it erupts later than the first, results from space loss following early loss of deciduous molar teeth. Extraction of the first premolar, to allow the second premolar to erupt into the arch, will give the best result. Only if the lower second premolar is excluded from the arch should it be removed.

Extraction of second permanent molars will provide little space further forward in the arch unless an appliance is used to retract the first permanent molars. Sometimes it is suggested that lower second molars should be removed to provide space for crowded lower third molars. The optimal time is shortly after root formation has begun, and for reasonable results it is important that the third molar is slightly mesially inclined. However, even in these favourable circumstances the result is unpredictable and it is usually preferable to have the crowded third molar removed surgically.

The Upper Arch

The key to a good incisor relationship is the occlusion of the upper canine with the lower arch. If the lower incisors are regular and the upper canines occlude in the embrasure distal to the lower canine, it should be possible to fit the upper incisors round the lower in alignment and with a normal overjet (*Fig. 47*). The major exceptions to this are where there is a mis-match in size between the upper and lower incisors (for example if the upper lateral incisors are peg-shaped the upper incisors will be spaced, while if the upper incisors are abnormally large they will be crowded), or where there is a marked dental base malrelationship which precludes the establishment of a normal incisor relationship. If the lower incisors are to be left crowded then the upper canines will have to be retracted beyond their correct relationship with the lower canines, otherwise residual upper incisor crowding or an increased overjet will have to be accepted.

Thus as a first step in treatment planning, space must be allowed to establish a correct relationship between the upper and lower canines (allowing for any change in lower canine position which will be produced by treatment).

The following discussion deals with malocclusions classified according to incisor relationship. As in the case of the lower arch, the discussion is based on the assumption that all permanent teeth are present, sound and in favourable positions. If this is not so, the treatment plan will have to be modified accordingly.

Treatment of the upper and lower arches must be co-ordinated. In Class I and Class II malocclusions, if extractions are planned in the lower arch, teeth will usually have to be removed from the upper arch at least as far forward as those from the lower. For example, if the lower second molars are to be extracted upper second molars or first premolars may be selected for extraction, depending on the amount of space required. However, if lower first premolars are to be removed it will usually be appropriate to extract upper first premolars, providing that the upper canines are favourably placed. This rule does not of course apply where a lower incisor or canine has to be removed.

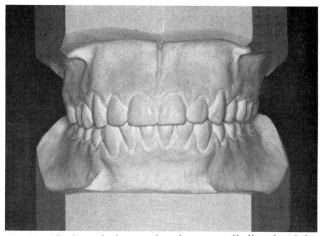

Fig. 47.—The lower incisors and canines are well aligned and the upper canines occlude correctly with the lower canines. It is therefore possible to obtain a correct relationship of the upper and lower incisors without crowding or spacing of the upper labial segment. Note that if there were a discrepancy in size between upper and lower incisors, or if there were a marked skeletal malrelationship, this rule would not apply.

In Class III malocclusions the rule is reversed: that is to say, if extractions are required in the upper arch, teeth at least as far forward should be removed from the lower arch unless it is spaced.

Class I Incisor Relationship

Treatment is directed towards relief of crowding and alignment of the teeth. The labio-lingual position of the upper labial segments is accepted and so stability is not usually a problem. However, it should be remembered that rotations are liable to relapse and that the

67

stability following treatment of a lingually placed incisor depends to a large extent on the presence of an overbite.

Where space requirements in the upper arch are small and lower extractions are not indicated, it may be possible to align the teeth without extractions. If the upper first permanent molars have drifted forwards, following early loss of deciduous molars, it will be necessary to retract them into the correct relationship with the lower molars. Provided that the upper third molars are present and of normal size, the extraction of upper second molars may be undertaken to facilitate the retraction of the first molars. The third molars will eventually erupt into a good contact relationship with the first molars.

The extraction of premolars is indicated where crowding is more severe. As in the lower arch, second premolars should be removed only if they themselves are crowded out of the arch. First premolars are the teeth of choice for extraction to relieve crowding in the incisor or canine regions. It is important that the canine is mesially inclined and it is usually advantageous for the extractions to be performed before the canine has fully erupted so that it will spontaneously drift into the extraction site. When this is done, care must be taken to ensure that forward drift of the buccal segments does not encroach on space required for the incisor teeth. Sometimes it is necessary to fit a space maintainer.

Occasionally the upper permanent canine is completely excluded from the arch and there is already a good contact between the lateral incisor and first premolar. If the appearance is satisfactory the simplest treatment is to extract the canine.

In a few crowded cases, where the permanent lateral incisor is palatally displaced and the canine erupts labial to it and adjacent to the central incisor, extraction of the lateral incisor itself may be considered. The appearance of a canine next to a central incisor is not ideal but alignment of the lateral incisor in these cases could involve quite extensive fixed appliance treatment.

Class II Division 1 Incisor Relationship

Ideally the skeletal pattern should be Class I or mild Class II and the upper incisors should be proclined so that, following overjet reduction, they are at an average inclination or only slightly retroclined. If the overjet is large or if the upper incisors are not proclined, simple tipping of the incisors will merely produce a Class II division 2 incisor relationship (*see Fig. 45*) which may well be both aesthetically unsatisfactory and traumatic. These patients require orthodontic treatment with fixed appliances.

The labio-lingual position of the upper incisors will be altered during treatment and it is important to assess whether they will be stable following retraction. Provided that the inner surface of the

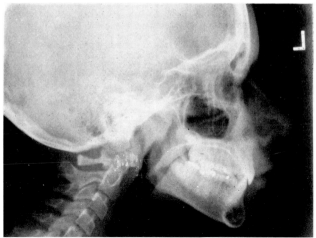

Fig. 48.—A treated Class II division 1 case. The retraction of these upper incisors will be stable because their position is controlled by the lower lip.

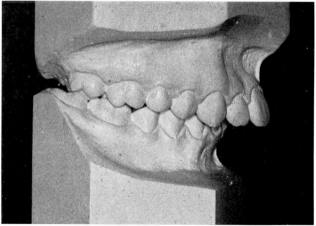

Fig. 49.—In this Class II division 1 malocclusion the lower arch is full premolar width distal to the upper. The lower arch is well aligned. Extractions will be required in the upper arch. In this case first premolars were removed.

lower lip covers the labial surface of the upper incisor edges (Fig. 48), the overjet should be stable.

Usually, prior to overjet reduction, overbite reduction is necessary. Stability of overbite reduction depends on stability of overjet reduction, and on the inter-incisor angle. If this angle is too wide (see p. 13) the overbite will deepen following treatment.

69

In a few cases, a Class II division 1 incisor relationship is associated with a normal buccal segment relationship with the upper canines occluding in the correct relationship with the lower arch. If there is no crowding in either arch these cases can be treated without extractions.

Where the buccal segments are in a mild Class II relationship and where there is no buccal segment crowding, retraction of the upper buccal segments into a normal relationship with the lower arch will provide space for reduction of the overjet.

In more severe cases where the upper canines have to be retracted by more than 3 millimetres (*Fig. 49*), or where lower premolars are to be extracted, removal of upper first premolars is normally indicated. If most of the extraction space is required for overjet reduction and relief of crowding, extra-oral anchorage should be used to prevent forward drift of the buccal segments during appliance treatment.

Class II Division 2 Incisor Relationship

In many cases, retroclination of the upper central incisors is not severe and the overbite is not likely to be traumatic (*Fig.* 50). Treatment planning should be based on an acceptance of the existing position of the upper central incisors. Space will frequently be required to accommodate the lateral incisors or to relieve crowding elsewhere in the arch.

Where space requirements are mild, and no lower extractions are planned, retraction of the upper buccal segments may be the most satisfactory method of treatment. As in Class II division 1 cases, the upper first permanent molars must not already be inclined distally. Extraction of upper second permanent molars may be indicated if third molars are present and of good size. On the other hand, if crowding is more severe or if lower premolars will have to be removed, the extraction of upper first premolars will usually be necessary.

If the overbite is so deep that there is the risk of periodontal damage (*Fig. 51*) or if the retroclination of the upper incisors is aesthetically unacceptable, fixed appliance treatment will be required to move the upper incisor apices palatally while maintaining the existing labio-lingual position of the crowns. Only by reducing the inter-incisor angle in this way can stability of overbite reduction be assured.

Class III Incisor Relationship

Only Class III malocclusions associated with a Class I or mild Class III skeletal pattern are amenable to orthodontic treatment. If the Class III skeletal pattern is at all severe, there is no hope of correcting the incisor relationship by appliances and orthodontic treatment is limited to relief of crowding and alignment of teeth. In many of

70

these patients it is the relative mandibular prominence which is unacceptable, and if treatment is to be undertaken it must be surgical.

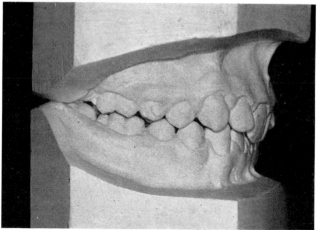

Fig. 50.—There is a mild Class II division 2 incisor relationship. The overbite is deep but not traumatic. The position of the upper central incisors should be accepted and treatment directed to aligning the lateral incisors which are slightly crowded.

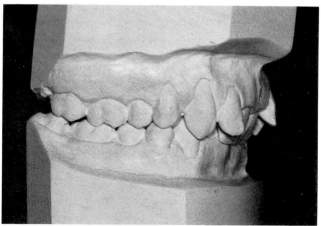

Fig. 51.—A severe Class II division 2 malocclusion. The upper incisors are markedly retroclined and the overbite is deep and potentially traumatic. Treatment is complex and fixed appliances will be required.

In mild cases where the patient can retract the mandible to obtain an edge-to-edge incisor relationship and where there will be an overbite following upper incisor proclination, appliance treatment to correct the incisor relationship may be possible. However, if the

71

upper incisors are already markedly proclined, further labial movement with an appliance is contra-indicated.

In the crowded upper arch extractions will be required. Many of these cases have a short upper dental base and the first permanent molars are distally inclined. This means that extraction of premolars, usually first premolars, is indicated.

Where the lower incisors are at all crowded, extraction of lower first premolars may be undertaken in the hope that the lower incisors will drop back slightly. However, any spontaneous movement of this sort will be minimal and the extraction spaces will not usually close completely. If a lower fixed appliance is used, it is often possible to retract the lower labial segment by a small amount but this will not be stable unless there is a definite overbite following treatment.

CONCLUSION

WITH careful diagnosis, treatment planning and timing of treatment, and by using removable appliances it is possible for the dental practitioner to obtain good results in those patients with simple malocclusions who form the majority of cases requiring orthodontic treatment. The dental practitioner will be wise to confine his attention to cases where the dental base relationship and soft tissue pattern are favourable and where the teeth can be tipped into the correct positions. Attempts to treat with simple appliances the more severe cases will only too often produce another malocclusion which is no more satisfactory, functionally or aesthetically, than the original. These difficult cases should, where possible, be referred for treatment to an orthodontic specialist, although he too is limited in what he can achieve by adverse dental base relationships and soft tissue patterns.

GLOSSARY OF TERMS

Soft Tissues

Competent Lips — A lip seal is maintained with minimal muscular effort when the mandible is in the rest position.

Incompetent Lips — With the mandible in the rest position muscular effort is required to obtain a lip seal.

Anterior Oral Seal — A seal produced by contact between the lips or between the tongue and lower lip.

Posterior Oral Seal — A seal between the soft palate and dorsum of the tongue.

Teeth and Occlusion

Ideal Occlusion — A theoretical occlusion based on the morphology of the teeth.

Normal Occlusion — An occlusion which satisfies the requirements of function and aesthetics but in which there are minor irregularities of individual teeth.

Malocclusion — An occlusion in which there is a malrelationship between the arches in any of the planes of space or in which there are anomalies in tooth position beyond the limits of normal.

Centric Occlusion — A position of maximum inter-cuspation which is a position of centric relation.

Overjet — The DISTANCE between upper and lower incisors in the horizontal plane.

Overbite — The overlap of the lower incisors by the upper incisors in the vertical plane.

Complete Overbite — An overbite in which the lower incisors contact either the upper incisors or the palatal mucosa.

Incomplete Overbite — An overbite in which the lower incisors contact neither the upper incisors nor the palatal mucosa.

Anterior Open Bite — The lower incisors are not overlapped in the vertical plane by the upper incisors and do not occlude with them.

74

Labial Segments	The incisor teeth.
Buccal Segments	The canine, premolar and molar teeth.
Incisor Classification	A classification based on the incisor relationship in the sagittal plane (*see* p. 12).
Angle's Classification	A classification of malocclusion based on arch relationship in the sagittal plane (*see* p. 9).
Crossbite	A transverse discrepancy in ~~arch~~ TOOTH relationship. The lower arch is ˄wider _sometimes_ than the upper so that the buccal cusps of the lower teeth occlude outside the buccal cusps of the corresponding upper teeth. May also be used for total lingual occlusion of the lower buccal teeth.
Scissors Bite	A lingual crossbite of the lower buccal teeth.
Leeway Space	The excess space provided when the deciduous canine and molars are replaced by the permanent canine and premolars. The leeway space is slightly greater in the lower arch.
Primate Spacing	A naturally occurring spacing in the deciduous dentition, mesial to the upper canine and distal to the lower canine.

The Dental Bases, Mandibular Positions and Paths of Closure

Dental Bases	The maxilla and mandible excluding the alveolar processes.
Alveolar Process	The parts of the maxilla and mandible the development and presence of which depend on the presence of the teeth.
Dental Base Relationship	The relationship between the dental bases, with the mandible in the rest position, in any of the three planes of space.
Skeletal Pattern	The relationship between the dental bases in the sagittal plane.
Intermaxillary Space	The space between the upper and lower dental bases when the mandible is in the rest position.

Bimaxillary	Pertaining to both upper and lower jaws.
Prognathism	The projection of the jaws from beneath the cranial base.
Positions of Centric Relation	The relationships between the mandible and maxilla when the condyles are in retruded unstrained positions in the glenoid fossae.
Rest Position	The position of the mandible in which the muscles acting on it show minimal activity. Essentially it is determined by the resting lengths of the muscles of mastication and it is a position of centric relation.
Habit Posture	A postured position of the mandible habitually maintained either to facilitate the production of an anterior oral seal or for aesthetic reasons.
Interocclusal Clearance	The space between the occlusal surfaces of the teeth when the mandible is in the rest position or a position of habitual posture.
Freeway Space	The interocclusal clearance when the mandible is in the rest position.
Deviation of the Mandible	A sagittal movement of the mandible during closure from a habit posture to a position of centric occlusion.
Displacement of the Mandible	A sagittal or lateral displacement of the mandible as a result of a premature contact.
Premature Contact	An occlusal contact which occurs during the centric path of closure of the mandible before maximum cuspal occlusion is reached. This may result in either displacement of the mandible or movement of the tooth or both.

Cephalometric Points and Planes

Sella (S)	The midpoint of sella turcica (the pituitary fossa).
Nasion (N)	The most anterior point on the fronto-nasal suture.
Glabella	The midline point on the profile at the level of the inner ends of the eyebrows.

Point A	The deepest point on the maxillary profile, between the anterior nasal spine and the alveolar crest.
Point B	The deepest point on the mandibular profile, between the point of the chin and the alveolar crest.
Porion (Po)	The uppermost, outermost point on the external acoustic meatus.
Orbitale (Or)	The most anterior, inferior point on the orbital margin.
Frankfort Plane	The plane through porion and orbitale. Theoretically this plane should be horizontal when the head is in a free postural position.
Maxillary Plane	The plane through the anterior and posterior nasal spines.
Mandibular Plane	The plane tangent to the lower border of the mandible.

SUGGESTED FURTHER READING

RATHER than provide a list of scientific articles which might not be readily available to the dental practitioner, this section lists a small number of standard texts which contain comprehensive reviews of various aspects of orthodontic diagnosis. The works cited contain extensive references and so will lead the reader who is interested in a particular problem into the primary literature in the field. Although only one or two chapters in each book are commented upon, all are standard orthodontic works that repay more extensive study. Texts dealing with a particular appliance technique have not been listed as they are primarily of interest to the orthodontic specialist.

Graber T. M. (1972) *Orthodontics*, 3rd ed.* Philadelphia, Saunders.
*4th edition due in 1975.
> Chapter 2 gives a clear account of growth and development while Chapter 15 includes a very extensive account of serial extraction procedures.

Horowitz S. L. and Hixon E. H. (1966) *The Nature of Orthodontic Diagnosis.** St Louis, Mosby.
> Chapter 16 presents a realistic appraisal of the problems in the prediction of facial growth. Chapter 17 is a sensible discussion in classification and treatment objectives.
> * OP

Moyers R. E. (1973) *Handbook of Orthodontics*, 3rd ed. Chicago, Year Book.
> Chapter 6 on the development of the dentition and occlusion is especially recommended. Chapter 11 contains an excellent account of the problems of space analysis in the mixed dentition.

Salzmann J. A. (1974) *Orthodontics in Daily Practice*. Philadelphia, Lippincott.
> Chapters 13 and 14 describe orthodontic and cephalometric radiography. Chapter 15 provides a sound introduction to cephalometric analysis. Chapter 35, by Dr. K. Reitan, is an excellent modern survey of the tissue changes in orthodontic tooth movement.

Salzmann J. A. (1966) *Practice of Orthodontics*, vol. 1 and 2. Philadelphia, Lippincott.
> An encyclopaedic work of reference.

INDEX